HELP YOURSELF!

For over three-quarters of a century, the Bircher-Benner Clinic of Zurich, Switzerland, has been the center of nutritional treatment of diseases. Its staff of physicians and specialists has developed an internationally acclaimed program of meal planning, treatment, and physical fitness that is outlined in this series of outstanding health guides.

The Plan for Liver and Gallbladder Problems provides a necessary guide for the many who suffer from these painful and often disabling diseases aggravated by faulty diet, sedentary life, insufficient exercise, and constant nervous tension. Here is a thorough understanding of the liver, the gallbladder and their functions, plus varied and enjoyable diets and menus to restore good health and well-being.

ABOUT THE
BIRCHER-BENNER CLINIC

In the nineteenth century, Dr. M. Bircher-Benner wanted to establish a kind of clinic that had never existed before: a clinic that would take into account the whole man, both body and soul, not only the patient's disease; a clinic that would use an intelligent patient as a co-worker in a total therapeutic effort; a clinic that would use the total knowledge of modern medicine to support the "internal physician"—the autonomous healing forces and healing system of the body—and in every case make the healing effects of dietetic therapy and one's life-style the basis of a total health plan; a clinic that, in addition to eliminating immediate ailments, would bring about a new, tougher, more satisfying and creative health of body and soul for the patient.

The private clinic founded by Dr. Bircher-Benner in 1897 is still operated today for that purpose.

Bircher-Benner Nutrition Plan For Liver and Gallbladder Problems

A Comprehensive Guide With Suggestions for Diet Menus and Recipes

Translated by Klaus Musmann

By the staff of the Bircher-Benner Clinic:

Medical/Dietetic Section:
D. Liechti-v. Brasch, M.D.,
P. F. Boesch, M.D.,
S. Grieder-Dopheide, M.D.

Physiological/Chemical Section:
Alfred Kunz-Bircher, Ph.D.

Menus and Recipes:
Ruth Kunz-Bircher, M.D.
(head of the Bircher-Benner Clinic)

Edited by Ralph Bircher, M.D.

PYRAMID BOOKS 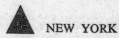 NEW YORK

BIRCHER-BENNER NUTRITION PLAN FOR
LIVER AND GALLBLADDER PROBLEMS
A PYRAMID BOOK

Copyright © 1972 by Nash Publishing

Pyramid edition published March 1977

ISBN: 0-515-04229-3

Library of Congress Catalog Card Number: 72-81865

Printed in the United States of America

Pyramid Books are published by Pyramid Publications (Harcourt Brace
Jovanovich, Inc.). Its trademarks, consisting of the word "Pyramid"
and the portrayal of a pyramid, are registered in the United States
Patent Office.

PYRAMID PUBLICATIONS (Harcourt Brace Jovanovich, Inc.).
757 Third Avenue, New York, N.Y. 10017

Contents

I. Introduction

Since the last world war, the number of men and women suffering from liver disease or from its consequences, that is, those who have a tender liver, has increased in staggering proportions. This is a consequence of infectious hepatitis which spread through Europe during the war years and which, after an apparent cure, has often left a permanent condition of hypersensitivity to foods and an overall weakening of physical strength. This condition is supported and maintained by the harmful effects of civilized living. A faulty diet, the sedentary life, insufficient physical exercise, and, above all, constant nervous tension affect the liver, its productivity and its rehabilitation after damage to a much higher degree than had been assumed earlier.

The liver patient is aware that the liver's performance depends directly upon its adjustment to food intake. He knows that dietary errors have immediate effects. Not only do they produce local discomforts in the liver area and in the digestive system, but they also lead to considerable disturbances in the patient's outlook, vitality, performance and mood as well as in his reactions to his surroundings. The patient is depressed after a setback, moody, withdrawn or irritable without meaning to be, and is not in the mood for any new undertakings. By and large the patient knows what foods to avoid to spare his liver, if he is a good observer and if he follows his own observations. But if he is generally unfamiliar with the composition and function of this organ which is of such vital importance to his life in so many ways, he may make mistakes all too often and will draw the wrong conclusions from his observations and thereby prevent the recuperation of his liver.

For this reason, the demand for a practical manual with a guide for the preparation and selection of meals has become ever more urgent in the last few years. We were asked to prepare such a guide because of our nutritional and dietary experience. This small book contains a summary of the conclusions which were derived from our decades of experience with patients and out-patients of the Bircher-Benner clinic. On the basis of this experience, the diet kitchen of the clinic, with the help of the medical staff, has created meals and menus which will provide the liver patient, the convalescent or the individual with a permanently sensitive liver with a varied, enjoyable diet that will make him happy. He will want to follow this diet willingly and it will help him to recuperate. We hope that we have succeeded in this endeavour.

Structure and Functions of the Liver

The liver patient or the individual with a sensitive liver should understand that the liver occupies a central position in the metabolism of the body. The liver accounts for 12% of the total metabolism of the body while its weight amounts to only 3% of the body's weight. Such intensive work takes place in the liver! One can guess from these figures what disturbances in the liver must mean for the health of the body. With its varied functions, essential to life, the liver is, indeed, of the greatest importance to man.

The liver organ consists primarily of a large number of small polygonal formations, the hepatic lobules which envelop the liver cells proper, blood vessels and the biliary ducts. They are interconnected through areolar connective tissue in which the blood vessels, the lymphatics and the nerves are imbedded. The cooperation of all hepatic lobules results in the effective functioning of the liver.

The liver is especially dependent upon an adequate supply of blood. Normally, the blood supply adapts itself to requirements of the liver, so that its blood content may rise fourfold if need be and, under certain conditions, function as a flood reserve for the entire body.

If the oxygen content is lowered due to circulatory disturbances such as a heart ailment or insufficient breathing and exercise, the capacity of the liver cells is impaired by a lack of oxygen. Gradually, a fatty degeneration develops in the liver lobules beginning in the center of the lobules. Their performance decreases and, tests indicate, the detoxification work of the liver slows down, bile production is reduced.

As the first organ to receive blood from the intestines, the liver selects, removes, synthesizes, and especially detoxifies the final products of digestion in the course of a few hours after each meal. The individual with a weak liver must be aware of the fact that the overall well-being of his body largely depends upon the liver's ability to do work well before new food can be taken in, and that incomplete detoxification leads to a backlog of unabsorbed food substances and unsecreted waste products, which tend to poison body tissues in many ways.

Normally, blood from the intestines leaves the liver with its burden removed and cleansed and flows through the *vena cava* toward heart and lungs to be recharged with oxygen.

Furthermore, the liver dispenses bile into the intestine to digest nutrients. Bile is a product of the parenchyma liver cells, a viscid liquid, yellow or greenish in color. When bile flows directly out of the liver, it is golden yellow and rather thin (A bile). If it is kept back in the gallbladder, it thickens to a dark black-green substance. This can be recognized very easily with the help of the duodenal probe: A thin rubber tube is inserted into the duodenum and collects the

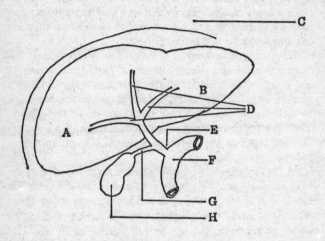

**Schematic Representation
of the Liver, Gallbladder and Bile Ducts**

A — RIGHT LIVER LOBE
B — LEFT LIVER LOBE
C — DIAPHRAGM
D — LUBERHEPATIC BILE
    PASSAGES

E — COMMON BILE
    DUCT
F — DUODENUM
G — CYSTIC DUCT
H — GALLBLADDER

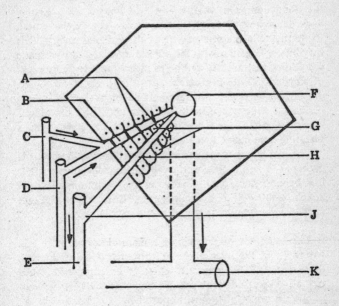

**Schematic Representation
of a Liver Lobule after Movill**

A — KUPFFER CELL
B — BLOOD CAPILLARY
C — BRANCH OF THE
       HEPATIC ARTERY
D — BRANCH OF THE
       PORTAL VEIN
E — COMMON BILE
       DUCT

F — VENA CAVA
       (INFERIOR)
G — LIVER CELLS
H — BILE CANALICULIS
J — HERNIG DUCT
K — BRANCH OF THE
       VEIN

bile. Through intake of a magnesium-enriched liquid the gallbladder is made to contract and releases its bile into the duodenum. Out of the tube will flow a thick, stringy dark substance (B bile), instead of a light yellow liquid. Primarily, bile consists of bile acids and pigments, and is very bitter. Together with the other duodenal and pancreatic secretions, it emulsifies and helps digest the fatty substances of nutrients. But if obstacles exist to prevent bile from passing through the discharging bile ducts into the duodenum, it will back up into the liver and enter the bloodstream. The result is a bile inundation of the body's tissues resulting in jaundice (see page 21).

The bile which is formed in the parenchyma liver cells is gathered in a thin network of capillaries, collected in larger interhepatic ducts and, finally, in the common bile duct which empties into the duodenum. Bile, when it is not needed immediately, is stored in the gallbladder.

The functions of the liver are manifold. The more one learns about the liver, the more one marvels and admires its versatility. One can only guess at its complexity since not all of its functions are known. The liver is, without doubt, an organ of utmost importance. It is situated in the upper part of the abdominal cavity, beneath the diaphragm. When distended, the liver pushes against the diaphragm, impairs breathing and pushes against the heart. The liver can also press against the stomach, the intestines, the bile ducts and the abdominal vessels. An infection in the area of the gallbladder, the common bile duct, the duodenum and the stomach can easily spread from one organ to another due to the open duct system. Thus, the harmony and interdependence of all parts must be kept especially in mind (as with any diagnosis), if one wants to obtain the desired goal.

A short summary of all known functions of the liver shall precede a more detailed description.

Secretions:

Bile production.

Metabolism Functions:

1. Carbohydrate metabolism. Conversion of carbohydrates from the intestines into glycogen.
2. Protein metabolism. Amino acid decomposition, urea and uric acid metabolism.
3. Fat metabolism. Desaturation of fatty acids through secretion of bile.
4. Mineral metabolism. Regulation of the acid-base equilibrium.
5. Water metabolism together with the endocrine glands and the kidneys.
6. Heat production. Vitamin synthesis of Vitamin-B group, D, A, K.

Storage Functions:

1. Vitamin storage.
2. Iron and copper storage (blood formation).
3. Storage of other elements for blood formation.
4. Glycogen storage of carbohydrates which are ready for use by the body.
5. Fat storage.
6. Protein storage.

Detoxification Functions:

1. Noxious food substances and bacterial poisons.
2. Destruction of inflammatory stimuli, infectious viruses and bacteria.
3. Regulation of sensitivity and defense mechanisms against injurious food and environmental influences, regeneration and restoration.

All of this is accomplished with the RES.† Although R.E. cells are found throughout the body, they are particularly well developed in the liver.

---

† Reticuloendothelial system.

Blood Clotting Functions:

1. Production of fibrinogen.
2. Production of prothrombin.
3. Production of blood platelets.

Regulation of Blood Volume:

Blood storage.

Hormonal Functions:

Probably present, but not yet clearly established in detail. For example, cooperative work with the adrenal glands and support of the ovary functions.

From this multitude, we will examine a few functions which deserve special attention.

Carbohydrate Metabolism

The liver stores sugar in the form of glycogen, which it synthesizes from starch, sugar, protein, and, if necessary, even from fatty substances, and releases into the bloodstream when the body needs sugar. Glycogen is not only stored within the liver cells but also used to protect these cells providing them with insurance and resistance similar to an accumulator. If the liver is low on glycogen, susceptibility to infection, poisoning and degeneration is greatly increased. It is therefore important that the liver receive an adequate supply of glycogen in the form of easily convertible carbohydrates (fructose) from fruits (fresh fruit, dried fruit, fruit concentrates) and especially from honey. For example, the blood receives glycogen from the liver for the maintenance and regulation of a stable blood sugar level. Without this process, extraordinary fluctuations occur in the sympathetic nervous system and in the performance of the endocrine glands, such as the adrenal glands, the pituitary gland, the ovaries, etc., which, together with the liver, maintain the blood sugar equilibrium. Such fluctuations are frequently observed in diseases of the liver. Blood sugar and sugar tolerance levels are therefore of great importance in the diagnosis of liver diseases. At times, diabetes may be simulated on the basis of a disturbed sugar storage function of the liver.

Protein Metabolism

From the amino acids of the diet's protein the liver synthesizes and stores body proteins. Thus, it maintains a stable protein level in the circulating blood. This is important, since blood protein, or plasma albumin, is the medium of transport for protein within the body. All body cells satisfy their needs from it. In a state of hunger, the liver gives up its reserves of protein and the body removes tissue protein to keep the blood level constant. The same self-consumption of the body takes place when the liver is diseased and fails in its protein production. In that case, protein concentration in the blood decreases slowly. To help such patients, one can attempt to equalize the loss with an enriched protein diet, or, better yet, make the patient temporarily independent from the liver's protein metabolism through injection of plasma albumin. A different view is taken by the Bircher-Benner therapy and, increasingly, also by other hospitals and physicians. In this view, an infected or degeneratively ill liver, which can no longer cope with its normal functions, is in need of rest so that it can recuperate instead of having to cope with an increased workload. Food consumption is limited and the amount of protein is kept low, and restricted to proteins which demand the least work from the liver. One such protein is casein which is derived from milk and, in its most easily digestible form, can be taken as low-fat cottage cheese, buttermilk or yogurt together with vegetable protein from green leaves and whole grain. Casein contains liver-protecting factors which work against fatty degeneration and dying of liver cells. Meat and other concentrated protein foods would mean a much greater labor for the metabolism of the liver than casein and are therefore completely omitted during treatment at the Bircher-Benner clinic. Time and again, we have observed that liver patients who did poorly on a diet consisting predominantly of meat, suddenly flourished on a lactovegetarian diet with plenty of fresh fruit. From a similar experience, other hospitals and physicians have prescribed a diet low in fats, rich in carbohydrates, with protein from cottage cheese and buttermilk, and little or no meat. In cases of acute liver disease, this has been more successful than an excess of protein. Such a diet has been used by the former Eppinger clinic in Vienna, the clinics of Heilmeier and Kalk, and of Badadrie in Canada. The latter recommends at most 25–30 grams of protein per day in the case of an acute liver infection, as compared to 130–200 grams of protein deemed necessary in the United States (and, until recently, in Europe).

Laboratory tests done at our clinic have shown that a meatless, low-protein diet rich in carbohydrates and fresh fruits and vegetables does not lower the blood's protein level in liver patients. On the contrary, it raises it in most cases. This proves, first, that the body does not become impoverished in protein, second, that the liver can recover on a frugal, lactovegetarian diet. However, the composition of the total diet is of utmost importance. Not only the supply of protein, but the proper distribution of various other nutrients in the diet of liver patients needs to be regulated. In summary, it can be said that 50–70 grams of protein are more than adequate and that, in the case of an acute liver disease, the supply of protein can be still further reduced to 25–40 grams. As little fat as possible should be consumed. It is to be completely avoided during an acute illness. Emphasis is put on fruit sugar from fresh fruits, vegetables and honey. Experience has shown that natural fruit sugar is a much better builder of liver glycogen than white refined grape sugar. The one-sided conclusions drawn from observing people on a starvation diet were based on an exclusive attention to protein content. A more realistic analysis would have considered all deficiencies—minerals, carbohydrates, vitamins, trace elements, and fresh foods.

Fat Metabolism

Since the liver produces bile it is directly involved with the digestion of fat. A diseased liver produces insufficient amounts of bile. Fats and fatty foods remain partially undigested and burden the intestines with decomposed products and bacterial changes, causing the familiar symptoms of fullness, bloatedness, constipation, and discomfort after meals. Fat intake must therefore be reduced in the case of liver ailments.

Aside from producing bile, the liver reconverts absorbed fats into neutral fats and releases them into the bloodstream for storage in the tissues. Excessive intake of fat, poisoning with substances such as alcohol, chloroform, phosphorus, or diabetes and pernicious anemia, may cause the liver to accumulate fat in its tissues. A fatty liver can no longer fulfill its tasks properly. It also becomes particularly depleted in glycogen and protein. If such a condition persists for a prolonged period, the distended, fatty liver will eventually shrink through degeneration of connective tissue and destruction of cells. It deteriorates into a scarred, deformed structure which can no longer be completely restored to its original condition. A less acute fatty degeneration of the liver may develop through impaired blood flow (insufficient oxygen supply) as mentioned earlier. Poor circulation due to lack of exercise, heart diseases with blood back-ups into the liver, pressure on the liver from intestinal gases, or advanced pregnancy may bring about such a condition. Stress from excitement, colds, sweating, excessive fatigue or psychic shock can also damage the liver cells in their functions and may lead to a tendency for fatty degeneration.

We can see from the foregoing that, beyond the immediate effects of the diet, general environmental factors influence the liver and its work. Thus, treatment of a liver patient should always include consideration of all circumstances, the individual's daily routine as well as his relationship to his surroundings.

Vitamin and Mineral Metabolism

The liver participates intensively in the vitamin and mineral metabolism, and one finds that in liver diseases nutritional deficiencies soon appear, such as dry, beriberi-like hands, changes in the mucous membranes of the mouth corners, in the mouth itself and in the entire alimentary canal, tendency to bleeding, brittle capillaries, disturbances in menstruation, decalcification of the skeleton, anemia and other problems, as well as difficulties in concentrating and thinking. The diseased liver needs a rich and balanced supply of vitamins and minerals for its recuperation. They should be provided primarily through a wisely chosen diet. However, temporarily, or during an acute stage of an illness, they may need to be injected directly into the bloodstream, thereby partially circumventing the work of the liver. This holds true especially for vitamins C, B_2, K, B_{12}, D, A and E. The attending physician will prescribe the correct vitamin supply. The liver is the organ richest in vitamins, and it is extremely sensitive to vitamin deficiencies. For example, with a deficiency of the B-complex, insufficient amounts of glycogen will be stored. Vitamin B_{12} together with liver extracts and easily reconvertible sugar from honey, fruit sugar (grapes, carrots, berries, and apples) work to prevent the destruction of the liver tissues. However, it should be stated emphatically that this marvelously complex organ, which accomplishes such tremendous feats and is exposed to so many damages, possesses an astonishing capacity for regeneration and self-healing, even after the most serious illness. Very often it can be completely restored through intelligent and consistent care. The liver, once diseased, decisively influences the mental and physical condition of the individual, and requires strict discipline in one's way of life and diet, but it rewards such discipline with concrete results in its recovery.

Thus, every effort is worthwhile. To facilitate understanding of the context in which the liver functions, the staff of the Bircher-Benner clinic has written this booklet.

Diseases of the Liver-Gallbladder System

The description of serious and acute liver ailments exceeds the scope of this booklet. A serious case of liver disease belongs without question and without exception under strict medical or even hospital care. In cases of mild, chronic disturbances, a thorough examination and advice from a physician is recommended, but the patient is able to speed up his recovery considerably if he has accurate information and a practical guide to carry out the medical advice.

Symptoms of Failing Liver Function

The healthy individual is unaware of his liver, and hardly knows where it is situated, or whether it functions properly. Not so the patient with liver complaints. He is familiar with a dull pressure and fullness in the right upper abdomen. He knows that he will be tired and unable to function for some time after each meal; that he must be careful at the onset of abdominal pressure, and cannot lie comfortably on his right side. He also knows that he is "sensitive" to a whole range of foods and must limit or avoid them altogether. When he exceeds his limits, unpleasant symptoms appear, such as flatulence, chronic constipation followed by sudden attacks of diarrhea with cramps, perceptible, often painful distension of the liver and waves of pain around the gallbladder. Lack of appetite or aversion to food may occur, usually in conjunction with constant nausea for one or more days. The tongue is coated and the corners of the eyes show a typical yellow discoloration. From bile which is entering the body's tissues, the skin, too, may be slightly yellow and may feel unpleasantly itchy. The head is heavy and dull and aches around the forehead and neck while waking up and frequently during the evenings. The morning awakening becomes a struggle. The eyelids seem to be swollen, hands and feet seem stiff, often accompanied by aching joints and calf muscles. The urine is a dark concentrate in the morning, becomes increasingly watery and clear and begins to flow in great quantities (a very typical disturbance of the mineral and water metabolism due to damage of the liver). Toward evening the liver patient becomes lively, or rather, he feels a nervous irritation which makes it difficult for him to fall asleep. His thoughts wander aimlessly in wild circles when quiet relaxation is needed. Creative individuals may find this wakeful state productive; others look for diversions, and, in a vicious circle, turn night into day, thereby placing the heaviest possible burden on the metabolism.

During difficult days, the patient will voluntarily limit his eating due to a lack of appetite and will reach for herb teas, fruit juices, dry bread, cereal purée or soup without fats. He will recuperate slowly with the help of such a diet until a new burden is placed on his system and a relapse occurs.

A rarely described, but conspicuous warning signal that all liver patients should be aware of is the following: a few days before a relapse occurs, that is, before the liver fails again, self-control and a healthy instinct for the right foods are apparently lost. Probably due to a change in gastrointestinal secretions, the patient craves the very foods which will clearly put a heavy burden on the liver. (Similar malfunctions occur during pregnancy.) It may be a sudden, overwhelming craving for chocolate, or for fat, spicy dishes, fat cheeses, bacon and deep-fried foods. If the patient gives in to these desires, a relapse becomes inevitable. If he recognizes and controls the situation, he can avert the relapse and his liver will be the better for it. A day of fasting with peppermint tea, fruit juice or fruit (especially grapefruit, berries, apples, and ripe oranges) and whole-grain crackers with honey will prevent such danger. In addition, sip bitter tea during the day to stimulate bile secretion; to relieve distension, apply heat in the form of hot compresses over the liver after each meal (it increases circulation); take a warm (not hot) bath before retiring; and finish with a Priessnitz compress (see page 28). Such drastic measures are certainly worthwhile since they prevent ten days of constant discomfort and feelings of illness.

The bowels, too, must be strictly regulated. It is best to start such a fast day by evacuating and detoxifying the bowels with an enema (1 qt. of camomile tea 2–3 times). Then, for the next 7–14 days one should take 1–2 glasses of mineral water every morning before breakfast. (For additional measures to stimulate bowel movement naturally, see the section on hepatitis).

If relapses occur over several years, far-reaching complications will develop. A strictly regulated diet and daily routine are necessary; artificial remedies and short-term treatments at spas cannot effect a lasting recovery.

Moreover, the following complications may arise: emaciation, chronic colitis, possibly migraine, inflammation of the gallbladder and formation of gallstones, colic, and periodic attacks of jaundice. The patient's personality change may overshadow family life. Lack of initiative, distrust and mental depressions, defeatism and suppressed anger are the greatest enemies of a harmonious coexistence in small and large groups of people. Finally, there is the danger of acute liver failure when a protracted liver disease remains untreated over a period of years.

Infectious Hepatitis

Although hepatitis is usually manifested by jaundice, the latter may appear in conjunction with other liver and gallbladder diseases as well. Moreover, hepatitis is not necessarily connected with jaundice.

Hepatitis is an infectious disease which breaks out with acute symptoms after an incubation period of several weeks or months.

The characteristics of the disease are: fatigue, dullness, depressions, and a noticeable lack of appetite with sudden, inexplicable cravings. Frequently, there is an uncommon, very pronounced constipation.

The disease breaks out with fever and a distinct general feeling of illness, often accompanied by respiratory infections. In a few days it develops into light to heavy jaundice, marked by discoloration of the eyes and skin, severe itching, paralyzing weakness, fainting spells while standing and, in serious cases, a toxic coma. Such patients need bedrest and medical care at the first sign of fever, since serious complications can arise which demand immediate preventive measures. Thus, the following remarks will be confined to diet and treatment in general.

Infection of the liver tissues and bile ducts causes bile to be pushed back into the bloodstream, and, partially or completely, prevents its release into the intestine, where it is needed for the digestion of fat. Therefore, fat must be completely avoided in cases of jaundice. When the condition improves and bile is present again in the intestine, fat can be given in carefully calculated amounts. It should be easily digestible, unheated as nut butter, cold-pressed olive oil, fresh butter, and small amounts of fresh cream.

In the first stage of the illness, when all food is rejected, serve warm herb teas such as peppermint, camomile, seed or bitter teas. The tea can be sweetened with honey, or honey may be served in small amounts diluted with water. Diluted lemon juice with or without tea is also permitted. Grapefruit juice or fresh berry juice by the spoon is also taken willingly. Red or black currants are especially good. Finely sliced apples or germ-free, seedless raisins can be given to chew on. Raw vegetable juices from carrots, beets, tomatoes and green leaves (pressed fresh, and served immediately) can be given also. Slowly, a few lettuce leaves, grated carrots and, especially, white or red radishes, chicory and dandelion may be included in the diet. But do not force the patient to eat. As soon as an improvement is shown, add whole-grain zwieback, crackers or dry bread, skimmed cottage cheese, buttermilk (later, yogurt), fat-free puréed cereal, and fat-free steamed vegetables. No cabbage and no legumes should be served. Aside from the diet, it is important to have regular bowel movements since the intestines tend to putrefy in the absence of bile. Toxic re-infection from the intestine is to be prevented under all circumstances. The feces have a gray clay color and cannot be confused with the light yellow, healthy feces from a diet consisting mainly of raw foods. As soon as the first sign of yellow appears in the feces, the height of the crisis has been overcome.

The bowel movements must be stimulated through camomile enemas, diet and specific additional substances. Recommended are abundant fresh foods, whole grains, and sour milk products; linseed cream (see recipe no. 39b) added to fruit juices or plain (2 cups a day), or 2–3 tbsp. of linseed flakes with muesli, fruit juices, or buttermilk; before each meal 1 tbsp. psyllium seeds, soaked in warm water for 1/2 hour (2–3 tbsp. daily). These are all natural products which stimulate the intestine without mechanical or chemical irritation.

Therapeutic Salts are also suitable to regulate bowel movement in a non-irritating natural way. Take 1 heaping tsp. 1/2 hour before every meal and, if needed, another 1–2 tsp. in the evening. The dosages are to be adjusted to individual requirements.

Mineral salt (Karlsbader Salz) should only be taken when prescribed by a physician. It is an excellent remedy to cleanse bile ducts and intestines, but, if taken in excessive dosages or for a long period of time, it can easily become an irritant and may disturb the mineral balance.

Mineral water works mildly and naturally and may be taken when needed or alternately with the above remedies. Drink 1 glass in the morning on an empty stomach, lukewarm, while walking.

Liver Cirrhosis

As stated earlier, cirrhosis develops from the fatty liver through increased toxicity and degeneration sustained through years of damage to the liver tissues and through incompletely healed infections. Massive scarring occurs with loss of the functioning liver tissues.

The causes are chronic tropical diseases, continuous consumption of alcohol, certain venereal diseases, liver infections, nutritional deficiency or overeating. In the advanced stage, the liver obstructs blood flowing from the intestines. Hyperemia develops in the intestine and abdomen, with hemorrhoids, varicose veins on the esophagus, accumulation of water in the abdomen and, possibly, dropsy. Increasingly, in the late stage, jaundice occurs. This is a very serious illness. Clearly, the still functioning liver tissues are in need of the utmost consideration and require a careful diet. Mistakes must be avoided under any circumstances. The liver should be kept warm. Bile secretion should be stimulated gently through bitter teas, certain mineral waters, and radishes. In addition, strict control of bowel movements, as described in the section on hepatitis, is necessary.

The mineral balance, disturbed through the loss of water, must be regulated with a careful raw-food diet and an adequate supply of vegetable broth. Carbohydrates should come from honey, fresh and dried fruits, whole-grain products (as grains, flakes, breads, and cereal soups) and simple potato dishes, proteins from cottage cheese, yogurt, buttermilk and soybean products in addition to the valuable protein from leafy vegetables and whole grains. Yeast extracts can be added in small amounts. Little milk should be given. The sources for fat are small amounts of fresh butter, yogurt, olive oil, nut butter and thin almond milk. No heated fats should be given. This diet plan follows essentially the menu under low-fat diets (see menu, page 39).

Diseases of the Gallbladder

The gallbladder functions as a special reserve system, and its malfunction through illness creates an added burden for the liver. Hence, it needs to be considered in the diagnosis. A gallbladder infection (in serious cases, suppuration) generally develops slowly, but it flares up acutely when the organism is overburdened or particularly exhausted. In most cases, the infection originates through bacteria in a chronically constipated intestine which is inflamed from overeating or a faulty diet. Since the infection can easily spread to the bile ducts of the liver, immediate and intensive care is essential. Similarly, full attention must be given to the intestine and its bacterial environment in order to exclude this source of infection in the future.

For all liver and gallbladder diseases, the treatment of the intestines is an essential factor. Constipation as well as diarrhea are signs of chronic gastrointestinal illness. More often than not, years of constipation have preceded it, followed by chronic diarrhea which is an infection of the large intestine. Over the years, this condition causes the stomach and intestine to lose their ability to properly select and reabsorb nutrients. Instead, they empty their contents explosively and loaded with infectious elements. The acid production of the stomach and the digestive juices of the duodenum and the pancreas decline.

A well-regulated intestine should be emptied 2–3 times daily. Stools should be soft and formed and should be released without cramps. A hard, dark stool indicates slow peristalsis and beginning putrefaction. Increased consumption of raw foods will often surmount such sluggishness without any other remedy. A stool which is the product of raw food has a light yellow color and cannot be mistaken for the clay-colored jaundice stool. The light yellow indicates active, fresh bile. Additional suggestions regarding bowel movement can be looked up in the section on hepatitis.

The gallbladder infection requires an accurate, detailed diagnosis. Pathogenic agents must be isolated and disinfected. Infected bile must be removed in order to clean the bile ducts. X-rays will have to decide in each case if stones have formed in the gallbladder, if growths exist, etc. Only a detailed knowledge of the individual case will provide a basis for treatment. Therefore, only general guidelines are given in the following.

Small amounts of food should be consumed, no sudden overburdening of the gallbladder system.

The diet should be low in fat (see menu on page 39), with plenty of herb teas and bile-producing mineral water.

Three main meals, and 2 snacks, consisting of herb tea, fruit juices, crisp rye bread, cottage cheese, soy milk, etc.

Chew and salivate well.

Regulate bowel movements.

Avoid excitement and sudden exertions.

Do not drink ice-cold drinks and alcoholic beverages since they cramp bile ducts and cause a relapse.

Avoid excessive cooling and overheating. The liver should be kept comfortably warm.

Ample body movement is suggested to stimulate the gallbladder, the bile ducts, the intestines, and breathing.

Massage connective tissues of the skin areas around the gallbladder to relax it and to stimulate flow of bile.

For oil treatments see page 38.

Gallstones

Gallstones develop mainly in conjunction with a chronic gallbladder infection through a thickening and crystallization of bile around infectious substances. But they may remain dormant, especially while the infection is under control. The feared gallstone attacks with raging pain in the gallbladder area come about when a stone is obstructed in the biliary ducts. Immediate medical attention and special medication are required. If possible, a massage of the connective tissues around the affected area is often helpful. During an attack, complete fasting except for a few sips of warm peppermint or camomile tea becomes necessary. Later, previously discussed recommendations for gallbladder infections should be followed. The gallbladder attack requires medical care.

A few words regarding treatments at spas: There are a number of excellent springs at home and abroad which can be of great assistance to the liver patient. But proper timing and duration must be determined solely by a physician. At the spa itself, a physician should prescribe the intensity of the treatment and the doctor should know the patient well. A spring water which promotes digestion too vigorously can have devastating consequences for the often existing colitis (infection of the large intestine). The daily amount of drinking water can be either just right and very helpful or useless and damaging.

Last but not least, drinking such spring water is not enough. Unfortunately, a large number of spas which may be ideal climatically as well as in the quality of their water, operate primarily as resorts with bars and restaurants. The administration is unaware that they could achieve a better reputation, and could promise their patients a much better chance of recovery, if they were to offer them a healthy diet and induce them to follow a therapeutic, daily regimen. Fortunately, a few exemplary spas exist in our country (Germany) which do consider this aspect of "guiding the ill," and thus, facilitate the physician's task.

Medication

There are a great many medicines, widely advertised and supposedly harmless. But we urgently plead not to obtain any medication without prescription. The variety of liver functions inplies any number of possible effects from medication as well as the danger of one-sidedness. Only a thorough knowledge of a given case history permits the selection of the right medication, if and when one is needed.

General Guidelines for Liver Patients

Daily routine. The liver must be given a daily rhythm by which to regulate its metabolism in order to regenerate itself.

Sleep. Long sleep before midnight. The violation of this rule on several nights often leads to a relapse in the case of sensitive livers. Early rising, and morning walks to stimulate breathing, bowel movement and circulation.

Nap. Rest for 1/2–1 hour. The liver area should be kept warm.

Walks. Two short walks should be taken during the day. For example, early in the morning and in the afternoon or in the evening before bedtime. Frequent long walks on Sundays but no strenuous hikes.

Breathing. Breathing is very important to stimulate the liver (oxygen supply). One should take a few breathing lessons, and then practice alone while walking or resting (5–10 minutes daily), preferably, in combination with massage to stimulate the liver region. While breathing, care should be taken to include the stomach muscles (liver massage).

Skin Care. Dry brushing and cool rubdowns in the morning. No cold showers after rising (shock); alternating cool and warm showers before or after the morning walk are preferable. A warm (not hot) bath in case of chills. During summer, 2–3 weekly cold compresses† should be given to induce sleep and to stimulate liver functions. Be sure to

† Priessnitz compress: Wet 1–2 broad, absorbent cotton cloths in cold water and wring dry. Fold lengthwise and wrap around the abdomen. Leave on over night or for 2 hours in the afternoon. The patient should feel completely warm.

warm up the body with a bath or walking before using the compress. Dry skin can be oiled with plant oil.

Exposure to Sun. Very helpful if used within reason. Head should always be in the shade when sunbathing. Length of sun bath should not exceed 5–15 minutes on each side. This should be followed by a cold wash and rest. No sun bath when fever, pain or jaundice are present, but fresh air is very good.

Diet. Fresh fruits and raw vegetables at the beginning of each meal. Small amounts should be consumed even with a large appetite. Eat simple dishes, rather than complex menus, to spare the liver. Fruits, salad and 1–2 cooked dishes should suffice. Refined or raw sugar should be used rarely. Eat only whole-grain bread. Preference should be given to green vegetables and ripe fruits, especially when the digestive system is sensitive. Three meals and a snack of 1 slice of whole-grain bread or cracker with honey or cottage cheese and herb tea are sufficient. The food should be well chewed and salivated.

Exercise. Do not overdo exercises. Slow training in the beginning. Rest when tired. Exercise the body evenly (breathing, circulation) with walking, swimming, and golf. Unwise choices are tennis, bicycling, rowing, climbing and horseback riding (unless it has been practiced for years) because they tax only parts of the body and involve nervous tension. Driving an automobile is not an exercise.

Vacations. Take frequent, short holidays to avoid long uninterrupted working periods. For example, every 2–3 months a week of vacation should be taken. On weekends, 1/2 day of bed rest and 1/2–1 day on a walking tour are recommended.

Emotional balance. Try to avoid, as much as possible, a tense atmosphere, demanding discussions, situations conducive to anger and tensions. By all means, avoid partying late into the night. Secure a daily hour of solitude when thoughts and feelings can be ordered and evaluated. Concentrate upon constructive and positive thoughts. This advice is of the greatest importance to the recuperation of liver patients.

Diet Table

CHRONIC LIVER DISEASES[1]	ACUTE LIVER INFECTION[2]	GALLBLADDER INFECTION AND GALLSTONES[3]
Fresh fruit: ripe, before every meal, whole or as juice	*Fruit juices:* with honey, diluted with mineral water, particularly grapefruit, orange, berry juice. Sliced apples	*Fruit juices:* as in col. 2, but generally undiluted
Dried fruit: especially raisins, figs, dates, prunes, bananas		*Dried fruit:* raisins, figs, bananas
Raw salads: without salt and with a little lemon and oil. Particularly green leaf salads, radishes (radish cure, p. 28), carrots, beets, artichokes, chicory, endives, dandelion	*Raw vegetable juices:* with a little lemon juice. Chew carrots or radishes or take as juice (radish cure, p. 28). Later, finely grated, non-fatty raw vegetables dressed with lemon and buttermilk. Masticate well.	*Raw vegetables:* as in col. 2, and mixed in blender. As salads: carrots, beets, lettuce, chicory, celeriac, artichokes. Masticate well
Honey: as sandwich spread, in herb or blossom teas, juices, and with muesli	*Honey:* plenty of honey dissolved in juices, tea, etc.	*Honey:* plenty of honey as in cols. 1, 2

Cereal grains: as whole grains, groats, flakes, purée, bread, sprouts, whole-wheat zwieback, crisp rye bread, any whole-grain products. Occasionally, soups (barley, rice, corn, wheat, rye, oats, buckwheat, millet). Chew well to avoid flatulence

Potatoes: with the skin, whole or mashed, with very little fat, or as raw juice before a meal

Vegetables: cooked without fat, but served with vegetable fat (if permitted by physician). Avoid cooked cabbage and legumes. Raw cabbage and raw sauerkraut juice are very beneficial, as are artichokes

Cereal grains: as purée or soup, cooked without fat, few whole grains, chewed well. Possibly crisp rye bread, flakes from millet, barley, linseed, wheat, oats

Potatoes: mashed, later whole with buttermilk, boiled potatoes without butter

Vegetables: cooked without fat. Selection as in col. 1

Cereal grains: as in cols. 1 or 2, depending on the seriousness of the illness

Potatoes: as in col. 1

Vegetables: Sautéed, small amounts of fresh butter. Otherwise, as in col. 1

CHRONIC LIVER DISEASES[1]	ACUTE LIVER INFECTION[2]	GALLBLADDER INFECTION AND GALLSTONES[3]
Vegetable stock: plenty of stock, low in salt, with yeast extract or soy seasoning. Prepare without fat	*Vegetable stock:* plain, fat-free	*Vegetable stock:* as in col. 1
Cottage cheese or cream cheese: plenty of such cheese, fat-free	*Cottage cheese:* low-fat, small amounts at first	*Cottage cheese and cream cheese:* plenty of such cheese, fat-free
Hard cheese: small amounts, low-fat		*Hard cheese:* small amounts, low-fat
Yogurt: low-fat and regular	*Yogurt:* made from low-fat milk	*Yogurt:* 1–2 glasses
Buttermilk: any amount	*Buttermilk:* any amount	*Buttermilk:* any amount
Cream: very small amounts, up to 1/4 cup, whipped—only with	*Cream:* none	*Cream:* as in col. 1

permission of physician

Butter: small amounts, only fresh, never heated, 1–2 tsp.

Butter: none

Butter: as in col. 1

Margarine: prefered over butter

Olive oil: none

Olive oil: plenty, possibly as a cure (see oil cure, p. 49)

Oil: cold-pressed, high quality sunflower, corn, linseed or thistle oil, if desired and tolerated

Nut butter: occasionally

Nut butter: as in col. 1

Soy bean products: permitted in any form

Soy bean products: as in col. 1

Liquids: herb and blossom teas of all kinds (see recipes), 1 cup per meal, 2–3 cups between meals. Also fruit juices with honey or mineral water. Diluted pure fruit

Liquids: herb teas, such as peppermint, Bitter tea, wormwood, seed tea, in sips, 3–4 cups per day. Mineral water to dilute fruit and vegetable juices and in sips

Liquids: as in col. 1. Mineral water as in cols. 1, 2, possibly more if on a special diet

CHRONIC LIVER DISEASES[1]	ACUTE LIVER INFECTION[2]	GALLBLADDER INFECTION AND GALLSTONES[3]
syrups, bile-stimulating juice diets (Spring diet), buckthorn juice, juniper berry juice, currant juice (red & black mixed), sauerkraut juice or finely shredded sauerkraut	up to 2 glasses a day (ask physician). Buttermilk or low-fat yogurt in slowly increasing amounts	
Mineral water, yogurt, buttermilk, very little regular milk (at most 1 cup; difficult to digest after jaundice)		
Eggs: if permitted, 2–3 egg yolks a week	*Eggs:* none	*Eggs:* as in col. 1 or more if on a special diet recommended by a physician

Restricted Foods

*Foods to be Limited
Generally:*

Butter: up to 1-1/2–2 tbsp.,
  if permitted by physician
Cream: up to 3/4–3 tbsp., if
  permitted by physician
Nuts and nut products: only
  if permitted by physician
Bread: no more than 2 slices
  a day (whole-grain). Instead, eat crisp rye bread,
  masticate well
Cooked foods containing
  milk products: oven-
  baked with cheese, pud-
  dings (1/2 milk,
  1/2 water)
Milk: at most, 1 cup of
  boiled or raw milk; yogurt
  or buttermilk are preferable
White flour, refined and raw
  sugar: only rarely and in
  very small amounts
Whole eggs: rarely and only
  for cooking purposes,
  never hardboiled

*Foods to be Avoided
Generally:*

Alcohol
Coffee: even caffein-free,
  since roasted products are
  not good
Black tea, mate tea
Heated fats of all kinds
Deep-fried, fried and baked
  goods, short-crust dough
Whip cream
Chocolate in any form
Fatty and sharp cheeses
Mayonnaise, rich sauces and
  gravies
Hard-boiled eggs
Meat and fish: only as rare
  exceptions
Whole milk: if tolerated,
  high-quality, raw milk and
  boiled milk are permissible
Unripe fruits
Ice cream, pastries, candy
Ice-cold or iced drinks and
  liquids

II. Spring and Fall Diets

Easily Digestible Oils: Corn oil, linseed oil, sunflower oil, and olive oil.

Margarine: Only cold-pressed fat from the health food store.

Linseed: 2–3 tbsp. of freshly cracked linseeds, soaked overnight and prepared as muesli with condensed milk or yogurt and fruit (see basic recipe, no. 1). This is a mild laxative.

Seasoning: Anise, caraway seeds, fennel, nutmeg, all locally grown herbs, yeast flavorings, cinnamon, cloves, curry and small quantities of paprika. Not recommended are mustard and pepper.

Salt: Sea salt and celery salt are preferred to the common cooking salt.

Mixed Vegetable Juices:

> 1/2 white radishes and 1/2 carrots
> 1/2 white radishes and 1/2 tomatoes
> 1/3 carrots, 1/3 celeriac, and 1/3 tomatoes
> 1/3 white radishes, 1/3 cabbage, and 1/3 tomatoes or carrots

Pure cabbage juice (rich in vitamin K) with a few
   drops of lemon juice or with 1/3 carrot juice
Potato juice from 1 raw, peeled potato of medium
   size. 1 sip before each meal or mixed with vegetable
   juice.

Mixed Fruit Juices: Any fresh berries with addition of
1/4–1/5 juice of black currants, grapefruit, orange, pitted
fruits (only when very ripe and sweet), melon, kaki, and
pumpkin.

Olive Oil Breakfast: 1–2 tbsp. olive oil, a few drops lemon
juice mixed with 1 slice whole-grain bread, cut into fine
cubes. Chew well after the oil has been absorbed by the
bread. Drink 1 cup peppermint tea. Duration: 2–3 weeks.

Oil Diet (morning, on an empty stomach after mouth
rinse and peppermint tea): 1 tbsp. olive oil with a few
drops lemon juice. 1 cup Bitter tea (see recipe no. 169) as
an after drink. Lie down for 1/2 hour on the right side
with a compress.

Sauerkraut Diet (morning, on an empty stomach): Raw,
finely cut sauerkraut (organic, from a health food store), 1
small plateful; chew well.

Horseradish Diet (according to Dr. Haemmerli, Zurich): Bring 1 lb. grated horseradish to a boil in 2 qts.
water, simmer for 5 minutes. Store for 24 hours in a glass
jar and squeeze out the juice. Drink 3-1/2 oz. of this extract 1/2 hour before the morning, noon and evening
meals. If the extract is too sharp, dilute with a little water.

Juniper Berry Extract: Drink after breakfast for 3 weeks,
according to directions.

Buckthorn and Radish Juice (morning, on an empty
stomach or at 4:00 p.m.): 3-1/2 oz. juice with a few drops
lemon juice and 1 tbsp. cream or 1-3/4 oz. juice diluted
with lemon juice and water. Vary according to individual
taste.

Mineral Water (such as Karlsbader Dinklbrunn, Muehl-

brunne, etc. 1 hr. before breakfast, on an empty stomach):
Drink 2 glasses of lukewarm mineral water while walking.
Duration: 3 weeks.

Haarlem Diet (evening): Take 1–2 capsules of Haarlem
oil. For 3 weeks; only when prescribed by a physician.

Bilifuge Diet: A concentrate derived from bitter herbs
(made by Lab. Plan in Geneva, Switzerland). 15 drops before every meal with a little water. Pleasant to take. Duration: approximately 4–6 weeks. To be taken preventively
before a heavy meal. Bitter tea can be used for a similar
effect.

Low-Fat Diet
To Protect the Liver

One Week for Every Two Months of the Year

Small amounts of vegetable margarine or cold-pressed
oils may be added to cooked foods before serving.

Breakfast: Muesli
Whole-grain or crisp rye bread with a little but-
ter, vegetable margarine or cottage cheese
and a little honey (opt.)
Herb tea or rose hip tea, sweetened with honey
For a change (instead of bread):
Cereal
Cream with yogurt and honey, *or*
Soya milk, almond milk or raw milk (if
tolerated)

Dinner: Muesli or grapefruit, *or*
Steamed rice and green salad
Whole-grain or crisp rye bread with a little
butter or vegetable margarine or cottage
cheese or soy spread, *or*

Rolls with cottage cheese, watercress, radishes
  and tomatoes, *or*
Potatoes in their skins with cottage cheese
Fruits, fresh or dried (raisins, dates, figs)
Herb tea or raw vegetable juice, *or*
Vegetable bouillon or soy soup

Snack: Herb tea or radish juice or vegetable- or fruit
(opt.)   juice, *or*
Yogurt, buttermilk, sour milk, soy milk

January-February

Lunch: †
1st day: Fruits
Raw Vegetables: celeriac, tomatoes, endives
  (possibly only 2 raw vegetables, one of which
  should always be a green leafy one)

Oat Groats Soup
Fennel
Caraway potatoes
2nd day: Fruits
Raw Vegetables: beets, fennel, Boston lettuce
Carrots
Apple sauce
3rd day: Fruits
Raw Vegetables: salsify, watercress, endives
Whole-wheat soup without cream
Celeriac
Potato snow
4th day: Fruits
Raw Vegetables: carrots, sauerkraut, Boston
  lettuce

---

† Lunch is the main meal of the day for all Bircher-Benner
diets.—ED.

Chicory
Soy spaetzli in tomato sauce
Fruit jello

5th day: Fruits
Raw Vegetables: radishes, tomatoes, corn salad
Spinach soup
Chinese artichoke
Bouillon potatoes

6th day: Fruits
Raw vegetables: broccoli, spinach, Boston lettuce
Soy soup
Swiss chard
Potatoes with tomatoes

7th day: Fruits
Raw Vegetables: celeriac, chicory, Boston lettuce
Sauteed Spinach
Rice
Oranges

March-April

1st day: Fruits
Raw Vegetables: carrots, fennel, endives
Salsify
Stewed pears

2nd day: Fruits
Raw Vegetables: cauliflower, Romaine lettuce
Tomato soup with farina
Fennel
Mashed potatoes

3rd day: Fruits
Raw Vegetables: celeriac, tomatoes, dandelion
Red beets

| | Noodles |
| | Stewed rhubarb |

4th day: Fruits

Raw Vegetables: beets, sauerkraut, Boston lettuce

Spring soup

Steamed Romaine lettuce

Potatoes with cottage cheese

5th day: Fruits

Raw Vegetables: radishes, spinach, endives

Artichokes in Vinaigrette sauce

Rice with chives

Stuffed apples

6th day: Fruits

Raw Vegetables: salsify, red cabbage, Boston lettuce

Whole-wheat soup

Chicory in tomato sauce

Potato snow

May-June

1st day: Fruits

Raw Vegetables: beets, zucchini, Boston lettuce

Vegetable stock

Kohlrabi with herbs

Potato snow

2nd day: Fruits

Raw Vegetables: celeriac, tomatoes, watercress

Zucchini

Polenta cooked in water

Strawberry whip

3rd day: Fruits

Raw Vegetables: carrots, cucumbers, Romaine lettuce

Chervil soup

Slices of celeriac (steamed, plain)

Rice with tomato sauce

4th day: Fruits
Raw Vegetables: kohlrabi, spinach, Boston
    lettuce
Romaine lettuce
Bouillon potatoes
Stewed rhubarb

5th day: Fruits
Raw Vegetables: radishes, zucchini, Boston
    lettuce
Whole-wheat soup
Taro stalks with herbs
Millotto mixed with carrots

6th day: Fruits
Raw Vegetables: cauliflower, watercress, Boston
    lettuce
Carrots
Potatoes in milk
Fruit jello (no. 154)

7th day: Fruits
Raw Vegetables: Boston lettuce, open-faced
    sandwiches with vegetable margarine and
    radishes, tomatoes, cucumbers, and water-
    cress
Spinach
Caraway potatoes
Strawberries with lemon

July-August

1st day: Fruits
Raw Vegetables: carrots, fennel, Boston lettuce
Soy soup
Steamed tomatoes
Whole-wheat noodles (no. 144)

2nd day: Fruits
Raw Vegetables: beets, cucumbers, watercress
Spinach or taro leaf soup

Cottage cheese potatoes

Berries with yogurt and raw sugar

3rd day: Fruits

Raw Vegetables: radishes, tomatoes, Boston
lettuce

Eggplant

Rice

Peach dessert

4th day: Fruits

Raw Vegetables: kohlrabi garnished with radishes, Romaine lettuce, Boston lettuce

Tomato soup

Steamed cucumbers with herbs

Potatoes in milk

5th day: Fruits

Raw Vegetables: cauliflower, watercress, Boston
lettuce

Carrots

Potato snow

Stuffed melon

6th day: Fruits

Raw Vegetables: beets, zucchini, Boston lettuce

Potato soup

Chopped spinach with raisins and pine kernels

Japanese rice with tomato sauce

7th day: Fruits

Raw Vegetables: carrots, cucumbers, watercress

Romaine lettuce

Parsley potatoes

Raspberries with lemon and raw sugar

September-October

1st day: Fruits

Raw Vegetables: celeriac, red cabbage, Boston
lettuce

Barley soup without cream

Zucchini with tomatoes
Bouillon potatoes

2nd day: Fruits
Raw Vegetables: carrots, cucumbers, Romaine
lettuce
Corn on the cob
Vegetable rice (leek, spinach, tomatoes)
Blueberry sweet

3rd day: Fruits
Raw Vegetables: kohlrabi, tomatoes, Boston
lettuce
Spinach soup
Celeriac and cottage cheese potatoes

4th day: Fruits
Raw Vegetables: white radishes, zucchini, Boston lettuce
Eggplant with tomatoes
Polenta
Melon with lemon and raw sugar

5th day: Fruits
Raw Vegetables: beets, cucumbers, Boston
lettuce
Vegetable soup
Taro stalks with carrots
Potato snow with vegetable fat

6th day: Fruits
Raw Vegetables: cauliflower, bell peppers, Boston lettuce
Farina soup
Baked tomato halves with parsley
Soy spaetzli without eggs

7th day: Fruits
Raw Vegetables: celeriac, tomatoes, spinach
Celery
Potatoes in milk
Orange jello

November-December

1st day: Fruits
           Raw Vegetables: white radishes, tomatoes, lamb's lettuce (corn salad)
           Fennel
           Millotto
           Orange mold
2nd day: Fruits
           Raw Vegetables: beets, chicory, Boston lettuce
           Oatmeal soup
           Spinach
           Caraway potatoes
3rd day: Fruits
           Raw Vegetables: salsify, red cabbage, endives
           Carrots
           Rice
           Stuffed apples with raisins
4th day: Fruits
           Raw Vegetables: carrots, white cabbage, Boston lettuce
           Tapioca soup with vegetables
           Romaine lettuce (steamed)
           Potato snow
5th day: Fruits
           Raw Vegetables: celeriac, red leaf lettuce, lamb's lettuce
           Steamed endive
           Noodles (no. 144)
           Farina pudding with raspberry sauce
6th day: Fruits
           Raw Vegetables: sauerkraut, tomatoes, chicory
           Rice soup
           Steamed celeriac
           Cottage cheese potatoes
7th day: Fruits
           Raw Vegetables: white radishes, Brussels sprouts, Boston lettuce

Mixed Vegetables: carrots, celeriac, spinach
with cranberries
Bouillon potatoes
Apple sauce

Fat-Free Diet (1 Week)
To Give the Liver a Rest

1st day

Breakfast: Grated apple with lemon and honey or meusli
prepared with buttermilk and honey

Whole-wheat bread or crisp rye bread with
honey

Possibly a few dried fruits

Herb tea or buttermilk

Lunch: Fruits

Raw vegetables: 1 carrot, 1 tomato, a few lettuce leaves. Eat whole or serve cut and
grated with a little lemon juice, low fat yogurt
and herbs

Vegetable stock without fat

Fennel with chives

Rice without fat and a little yeast seasoning

Dinner: Grapefruit with honey

Whole-wheat bread with honey

Cream of oat soup

Rose hip tea with honey or buttermilk

2nd day

Breakfast: As above for all subsequent days.

Lunch: Fruits

Raw vegetables: celeriac and fennel (no dressing), lamb's lettuce with lemon and herbs

Spinach

Caraway potatoes, nonfat

Baked apple with raisins, grapes and a little
honey

Dinner: Grated apples and bananas with lemon and a little honey

Bread or crisp rye bread with tomatoes

Dried fruits (dates, figs, raisins)

Rose hip tea or herb tea

3rd day

Lunch: Fruits

Raw vegetables: cauliflower, tomato, or tomato juice, Boston lettuce leaves

Cream of barley soup (without fat)

Steamed celeriac (plain)

Polenta, nonfat, with a few herbs

Dinner: Fruit salad with lemon and honey

Plain rice with baked tomato halves

Herb tea

4th day

Lunch: Fruits

Raw vegetables: carrots or radish juice, cucumber, watercress

Salsify (steamed without fat)

Potato snow

Dinner: Fruits, fresh and dried

Nonfat potato soup with many herbs

Whole-grain bread

Rose hip tea

5th day

Lunch: Fruits

Raw vegetables: white radishes or radish juice, celery, Boston lettuce

Nonfat spinach soup

Romaine lettuce (steamed, plain)

Whole-wheat noodles in tomato sauce with herbs (no fat)

Dinner: Fruit juice

Potatoes in their skin

Cucumber salad without oil or cooked carrot salad with lemon, salt and herbs

6th day

Lunch: Fruits

Raw vegetables: beets or beet juice, zucchini, spinach leaves

Artichokes in Vinaigrette sauce without oil

Potato snow with carrot sauce (steamed carrots blended with nonfat stock and a little flour)

Apple sauce

Dinner: 1 grapefruit

Rice vegetable soup

Crisp rye bread with honey or rose hip jam

Herb tea or buttermilk

7th day

Lunch: Fruits

Raw vegetables: radishes, tomatoes, Boston lettuce leaves

Nonfat vegetable stock

Steamed tomatoes, without fat

Japanese rice

Dinner: Fruit salad with lemon and raw sugar

Baked potato

Cooked beet salad with lemon

Cooked spinach with lemon

Herb tea or buttermilk

Note: 1/2 hour before lunch, 1 small cup Bitter tea. At 4:00 p.m. in the afternoon, 1 cup of peppermint tea or radish juice.

III. Recipes

Muesli

Apple muesli, as introduced by Dr. Bircher, has proved itself to be the best diet dish according to our long experience.

The originally added sweetened condensed milk is now usually—always for liver and gallbladder patients—substituted with yogurt and honey or pure fruit syrups as a natural sweetener. Refined sugar should be avoided. Yogurt is more easily assimilated, stimulates the digestion better and is less filling.

As a rule, tart, white-fleshed, juice apples are best. For example, Cortland, McIntosh, Rhode Island Greening. Northern Spy, Winesap, Jonathan and Gravenstein may be used.

The flavor of dry or tasteless apples, late in the season, can be improved by adding some freshly grated orange or lemon peel, orange juice or, at times, some rose hip purée just before serving. All recipes are for one serving.

1. Apple Muesli with Yogurt

1 tbsp. rolled oats
3 tbsp. cold water
1–1-1/2 tsp. lemon juice
3 tbsp. yogurt
1 tbsp. honey
1–2 tbsp. water, depending on the type of apple
1 large apple

Soak rolled oats overnight in water. Blend lemon juice, honey and yogurt into a smooth cream and add to oats. Wash apple, dry with a clean cloth, remove top, core and blemishes. Grate apple finely directly into the cream, stirring frequently to prevent discoloring. The grating should be done just before serving.

Instead of 1 tbsp. rolled oats, 1 tsp. rolled oats (previously soaked) and 1 tsp. whole grains or wheat germ may be used.

Wheat, rice, barley, rye, millet, buckwheat or soy flakes can also be used, as well as wheat flakes, possibly mixed with yeast flakes for vitamin-B enrichment. They are obtainable at health food stores.

Rolled oats or oatmeal must be soaked in water for 12 hours. Quick cooking flakes should not be soaked, but the quantity of water remains the same.

Whole grains must be soaked in water for 24 hours, then rinsed through a sieve in cold water and used either whole, coarsely ground or chopped in blender.

2. Muesli with Berries or Stone Fruit

(Especially rich in vitamin C. Use stone fruit only on physician's advice.)

3/4 cup strawberries (selected and well washed), *or*
Raspberries, loganberries, currants, blackberries (selected and well washed), *or*
1/2 lb. plums, peaches, apricots

Berries should be crushed with a wooden spoon or fork. For stone fruit, remove stones, chop up or reduce to pulp in electric blender. Preparation of cream as in recipe no. 1.

3. Muesli with Mixed Fruit

Strawberries and raspberries
Strawberries, raspberries and currants
Strawberries and apples
Blackberries and apples
Apples with finely chopped orange or tangerine slices
Apples and bananas
Plums and peaches or apricots, etc.

Preparation as in recipe no. 1.

4. Muesli with Dried Fruit

If necessary, muesli may be prepared from dried fruits (apples, apricots, and prunes). Wash 1/2 cup fruit per serving in cold water, soak in water for 12 hours and put the fruit through a mincer or blender. This purée should be added to the basic cream as in recipe no. 1.

Dried fruit should be of good quality without preservatives or bleaching agents, otherwise, troublesome gastric and intestinal disturbances may occur. This muesli is especially conducive to stimulate digestion.

5. Raw Banana Cream

2 tbsp. of soaked, cracked grains are finely ground in a blender. Add half a banana to the mixture, a tsp. honey and lemon juice, according to taste. Serve immediately.

Raw Vegetables

The following four principles should be observed in the preparation of raw vegetables:

Freshness

The best vegetables are sun-ripened, organically grown from one's own garden. Raw vegetables should be served immediately after preparation so that no wilting and loss of juice occur. The cut-up vegetables should not be exposed to the air for too long. They should be mixed with the dressing immediately.

Quality

Choose leaf and roof vegetables that are young, tender and of good color. They should not have been grown on excessively fertilized soil, but should have been fertilized with compost and be free of plant diseases. This is especially important for an invalid's diet.

Well-balanced Mixtures

Every raw vegetable dish should consist of root, fruit and leafy vegetables. A patient's diet, in particular, should always contain green leaves. The dressing which is used for the same vegetables should be varied.

Bright colors increase the beauty of the salad dishes and the pleasures of eating.

Garnishes of herbs, radishes and young carrots, etc. can be used effectively for more festive occasions, but not more than three raw vegetables should be served per daily meal. More variety can be offered during the rest of the day, as a multitude of vegetables at one meal may inhibit good digestion.

Thorough Cleaning

To get rid of worms and to avoid infections from coli-bacilli, one should follow very carefully the instructions given below. Organic vegetables and those grown without manure contain no worm eggs.

Cleaning Leafy Vegetables: With Boston lettuce, endive, Romaine lettuce, white cabbage, red cabbage, etc., separate leaves, remove brown and imperfect parts, and soak for 1 hour in salt water (1 handful of salt to 6 qts. water). Rinse several times, wash each leaf separately under the tap. Dry well in a wire basket or in a clean cloth.

Particular care should be taken with the preparation and washing of lamb's lettuce (corn salad), spinach, dandelion, watercress, Brussels sprouts and similar small leafy salads. Rinse several times, and remove any little roots and tough parts.

Cut chicory in half, remove outer leaves and wash well.

Cleaning Root Vegetables: Scrub celery roots, carrots, salsify, beets, radishes, kohlrabi with a brush under running water. Peel and put immediately into cold water to which salt and lemon juice have been added (1/2 lemon or squeezed-out peel to approximately 6 qts. of water) so that vegetables will not lose their fresh color.

Cleaning Vegetable Fruits: Tomatoes, cucumbers, zucchini, green and red peppers should be washed, peeled if necessary, and chopped.

Cucumbers should be peeled from the center to the ends. Cut off bitter ends. Tender cucumbers may be left unpeeled.

Use only young, tender zucchini for salads. Do not peel. Green and yellow peppers are less sharp than the red ones. Cut peppers in half and remove seeds, score thick parts and soak in water if they are too sharp.

Cauliflower, celery, leeks, fennel: Cut cauliflower into large pieces, cut off blemishes, scrape stalk lightly and put into salted water.

Peel celery, cut off tough parts.

Cut leeks in half, remove brown parts and wash under running water.

Cut fennel in half and wash.

All of these vegetables should also be put into salt water before washing.

Special Cleaning Methods

If any doubt exists regarding the cleanliness or freedom from bacteria of any vegetable or fruit (especially in southern and tropical countries and in case manure was used as fertilizer), the following cleaning methods should be observed:

1. To destroy worm eggs and insects, put vegetables into a diluted salt water solution (1 handful of salt to approximately 6 qts. water). The solution dissolves the

layer of protein by which worm eggs are attached. The vegetables are cleansed in subsequent rinsing.

2. Bacteria, colibacilli and fungi, which are not harmful to healthy individuals in northern regions, can be removed with citric acid or vinegar. The vegetables, particularly the leafy ones, should be left for 15 minutes in a solution of 2 oz. citric acid (available in drugstores) to approximately 1 qt. water. Rinse well under tap water. Save citric acid solution. It may be re-used 3 or 4 times.

3. Put cleaned root vegetables and vegetable fruits in a sieve and dip for 10 seconds into boiling water. This will free the outer layer of bacteria while the inside of the vegetable remains raw.

4. Vegetable and fruit juices can be virtually freed of bacteria by adding squeezed lemon juice (1/5 of the total quantity of juice).

5. To be protected from the danger of amebic infection, dip prepared vegetables into a chloride of lime solution (1/2 tbsp. to 1 qt. water). Wash again in boiled water to remove all traces of the solution.

Cutting up Various Vegetables

Boston lettuce, red leaf lettuce, lamb's lettuce, dandelion, watercress—leave whole or cut into half the largest leaves.

Romaine lettuce, endive, chicory—cut into 1/4 inch strips.

Spinach, leeks, peppers, celery, fennel—cut into very small strips.

Cabbage, white or red—shred finely.

Carrots, celeriac, beets, radishes, salsify, kohlrabi—grate with fine or coarse grater.

Cucumber, zucchini, radishes—slice very finely.

Cauliflower—cut florets and tender stalks very finely.

Cabbages, peppers, salsify, kohlrabi should be given at first only as juice if the patient is flatulent (see page 64).

Salad Dressings

6. Oil Dressing (For 1 serving)

1/2 tbsp. oil
1 tsp. lemon juice
1 tsp. fresh or 1/4 tsp. dried herbs

Mix all ingredients well.

7. Yogurt or Buttermilk Dressing (1 serving)

2–3 tbsp. yogurt or buttermilk
A few drops lemon juice
1 tsp. fresh or 1/4 tsp. dried herbs
Onion or garlic juice (opt.)

Whisk all ingredients thoroughly together.

8. Cottage Cheese Dressing

1 tbsp. low-fat cottage cheese
3 tbsp. buttermilk (approx.)
1 tsp. lemon juice
Fresh, finely chopped herbs

Whisk all ingredients together. Especially good with artichokes and corn.

Suggested Dressings for Raw Vegetable Salads

Items marked with an asterisk are especially good for liver patients.

9. Boston Lettuce

Do not cut. Use oil dressing.

10. Red Leaf Lettuce

Do not cut. Use oil dressing.

11. Endive

Cut into 1/2 in. strips. Use oil dressing, basil, marjoram.

12. Romaine Lettuce*

Cut into 1/2 in. strips. Use oil dressing.

13. Lamb's Lettuce

Do not cut. Use oil dressing.

14. Cress

Do not cut. Use oil dressing.

15. Spinach

Cut into 1/2 in. strips. Use oil dressing, peppermint, borage.

16. Cabbages: white sauerkraut,* Brussels sprouts, Savoy, Chinese cabbages

Shred finely into small strips. Use oil dressing, lovage, thyme, caraway, savory.

17. Tomatoes

Slices or dice. Use oil dressing, basil, dill, thyme.

18. Cucumbers

Slice finely. Use oil dressing, dill, borage.

19. Fennel*

Slice finely and chop. Use oil dressing.

20. Peppers*

Cut in fine strips. Use oil dressing.

21. Radishes:* large red or white

Slice or grate. Use oil dressing.

22. Radishes,* small red

Slice. Use oil dressing.

23. Celery

Slice finely. Use oil dressing.

24. Squash or Zucchini

Slice finely or grate coarsely. Use yogurt, buttermilk or cottage cheese dressing, dill, basil.

25. Carrots*

Grate finely. Use yogurt, buttermilk or cottage cheese dressing, marjoram, chervil.

26. Celeriac

Grate finely or coarsely. Use yogurt, buttermilk or cottage cheese dressing, caraway, lovage, thyme.

27. Beets*

Grate finely or rough. Use yogurt, buttermilk or cottage cheese dressing, caraway, lovage, thyme.

28. Cauliflower

Separate florets, grate stalks. Use yogurt, buttermilk or cottage cheese dressing, basil, marjoram.

29. Chicory

Cut into 1/2 in. strips. Use yogurt, buttermilk or cottage cheese dressing, thyme, tarragon.

30. Jerusalem Artichokes

Grate. Use yogurt, buttermilk or cottage cheese dressing, thyme, lemon balm.

31. Kohlrabi

Shred and chop finely. Use yogurt, buttermilk or cottage cheese dressing, thyme, lovage.

32. Red Cabbage

Shred or cut finely. Use yogurt, buttermilk or cottage cheese dressing, some grated apples.

33. Artichokes*

Halve, cut out heart. Use yogurt, buttermilk or cottage cheese dressing, caraway, lovage.

Finely chopped onions, chives and possibly parsley or their juices can be added to all salads according to taste.

34. Sprouted Cereal Grains

(Especially high in vitamin E and the vitamin B group. Good source of energy.)

Use wheat, rye, oats, barley.

1st day
Evening: Wash grains in sieve under running water and put into a small bowl. Cover with water. Keep at room temperature near oven.

2nd day
Morning: Rinse and spread out to dry on flat plate. Keep at room temperature near an oven.

3rd day
Morning: Rinse and spread out to dry on a plate.

Evening: Return to bowl and cover with water. Keep at
room temperature, near an oven.

The grain should have developed 1/2–3/4 inch sprouts.

35. Sauerkraut

An especially valuable raw vegetable particularly during
the winter, sauerkraut is easier to digest raw than cooked.
If it is cooked, its taste and digestibility can be improved
by adding finely cut fresh sauerkraut. (See also, Sauerkraut
Diet, page 38.)

36. Sauerkraut Salad *(Stimulates bile and disinfects)*

Loosen sauerkraut and cut up. Mix with a few caraway
seeds or ground caraway. Add 3–4 crushed juniper berries,
some finely cut onion, and 1/4 shredded apple. Add the
juice of a lemon and 1 tsp. olive oil. Any raw root vegetable
is recommended as an addition.

Juices

Juices are raw foods in liquid form, intended as an additional enrichment and in cases where roughage must be
avoided or in cases of liver and gastrointestinal illnesses
(see Diet Table, page 30).

However, one should not forget that whole food is always more wholesome and that it cannot be replaced permanently by juice. A return to fruits and raw vegetables
is recommended as soon as permitted.

In general: For cleaning, see the chapter on "Salads and
Raw Vegetables." Many extractors are available for prepar-

ing fruit and vegetable juices, from small hand models to large, electric ones. Fruit and vegetables must be cut up if a hand model is used. Apples, pears and all root vegetables should be finely grated, and leafy vegetables and herbs should be finely chopped.

Many high-quality grape, fruit and vegetable juices can be obtained in health food stores for those who do not have the facilities to make their own juice.

37. Fruit Juices

Serve immediately after squeezing. Delay causes loss in value.
a) Unmixed Fruit Juices (without any addition):
   Oranges, tangerines, grapefruit, apples, pears, grapes, strawberries, loganberries, currants, raspberries, peaches, apricots, and plums.
b) Mixed Fruit Juices:
   Oranges, tangerines, grapefruit, persimmon or berry juice with apple juice
   Berry juice with peach, apricot or plum juice
   Bananas, mashed and whisked, with orange, berry, peach, and apricot juice.

Depending on prescription, add a few drops of lemon juice, or lemon juice and 1 tbsp. yogurt, or lemon juice and 1 tbsp. buttermilk per glass.

38. Vegetable Juices

Served immediately, they have a high mineral and vitamin content. Each juice has its own special value.
a) Unmixed Vegetable Juices:
   Tomatoes, carrots, beets, white radishes, cabbage, celery, potatoes, all leaf, root and tuberous vegetables.

b) Mixed Vegetable Juices:
The best mixtures are, in our experience: Carrots, to-
matoes, and spinach (in equal proportions)
Tomatoes and carrots
Tomatoes and spinach.

Other mixtures and cocktails can be combined to taste.
For a change, add to the mixture before extracting, some
sorrel, tender nettles, chives, parsley, onions, tender young
celery leaves or roots and other herbs. Juice made from
raw potatoes helps against cramps.

Add, per glass, a few drops of lemon juice, 1 tbsp.
yogurt, a little honey or pure fruit syrup or 1 tbsp. buttermilk.

Other leafy vegetables or salads which may be added are
white cabbage, kale, Boston lettuce, endives, lamb's lettuce,
and dandelion.

In spring, tender nettles, sorrel and dandelion juice may
be taken to cleanse the blood. Cabbage juice is helpful for
liver and stomach ailments.

39. Cereal Purée as an Addition to Juices

One third cereal purée may be added to raw juices to
neutralize tart fruit flavors.

a) Rice or Barley Purée
    (Constipating)
        1 heaping tsp. rice or barley flour
        1 cup water

Mix flour with cold water and bring to a boil. Cook for
five minutes, stirring constantly. Allow to cool.

b) Linseed Purée
    (Slight laxative.)
        1 tbsp. linseed
        1 cup water

Wash linseed, and boil in water for 10 minutes. Strain and allow to cool.

Varieties of Milk

40. Almond Milk

(Rich in vegetable protein, mucilaginous, soothing. For liver patients only if fat is permitted.)

- 1 tsp. almond purée
- 1 tsp. honey
- 3/4 cup water, *or*
- 3/4 cup water and 1/4 cup fruit juice (will produce slight thickening)

Mix almond purée and honey together with whisk. Add water drop by drop while stirring well.

41. Almond Milk from Fresh Almonds

(Especially easy to digest.)

- 1-1/2 tbsp. peeled almonds
- 1 tsp. honey
- 1 cup water

Chop almonds and liquefy all ingredients in blender.

42. Sesame Milk

(Only when well recovered, since it is very rich in fats.)

> 1 cup water
> 1 tsp. sesame purée
> 1 tsp. lemon juice
> 1 tsp. raw sugar or honey

Mix sesame purée and sugar or honey with whisk and add water drop by drop (cold or warm, depending on taste).

43. Pine Kernel Milk

(Very rich in easily digestible fat and vegetable protein.)

> 1 tbsp. washed pine kernels
> 1 tsp. honey
> 3/4 cup water

Prepare like Almond Milk, recipe no. 41.

44. Soy Milk

(High-quality vegetable protein.)

Made from Soyamel or other commercially available soy powders, lightly sweetened, sour or unsweetened. Follow directions on package.

45. Yogurt, I

Yogurt made from skimmed milk is the purest, most effective and most easily digestible milk protein. It stimulates the digestion. The simplest home method known to us to make yogurt is with an electric yogurt maker (available in health food stores). The manufacturer's directions should be followed closely.

46. Yogurt, II

1 qt. milk
1 tbsp. yogurt

1. Bring milk to a boil and cool to 100°F.
2. Whisk yogurt together with milk.
3. Pour into a glass receptacle.
4. Cover with cheese cloth and a tight-fitting lid.
5. Leave in a uniformly warm place for 24 hours.
6. Keep refrigerated until use.

Note: Health food stores have commercially available, high-quality yogurt. For certain diets, low-fat yogurt, made from skimmed milk, is preferred.

Buttermilk contains no fat, but all the minerals, proteins and carbohydrates of milk (see Diet Table for specific uses).

Vegetable Fats and Oils

The amount of fat intake depends on the physician's advice and the patient's tolerance; meals can also be prepared free of fats. We use vegetable fats and oils (cold-pressed) exclusively for liver patients. The oil is never heated.

Cold-pressed vegetable margarine and fats:	Vegetable fat emulsions from naturally solid fats such as coconut or palm kernel oil in conjunction with a high proportion of liquid oils and germ oils, especially sunflower oil.
Nut and almond butter:	Delicate, nut flavor; of many uses for kitchen and table, particularly for diets. Add, instead of fresh butter, to vegetables, potatoes, rice and noodles.
Cold-pressed sunflower oil, germinated corn oil, linseed oil, olive oil:	Organically processed, rich in highly unsaturated fatty acids. Due to their purity, these fats are biologically very valuable and more easily digestible by most people than heated butter.

Soups

Soups can be prepared without fat in the case of fat-free diets. Vegetables in soup recipes marked with an asterisk are to be steamed briefly in a small amount of fat-free vegetable stock. Add 1 tsp. vegetable fat or oil to the serving bowl (except with a strict fat-free diet).

47. Vegetable Stock

Choose vegetables in season. For example, celery roots, carrots, a little cabbage or kohlrabi, leeks, tomatoes. Tough but sound vegetable parts may also be used as well as potato peels. (This recipe serves 4, all others serve 1.)

1 onion
2 carrots
1 small celery root
Cabbage
1/2 bay leaf
Taro leaves
1 large or 2 small leeks
3–4 qts. cold water
Lovage, basil or other fresh or dried herbs

*Halve unpeeled onion and brown cut surface in vegetable fat. (Omit this step for liver patients on a fat-free diet.) Cut vegetables into small pieces, add to the onion, cover and sauté briefly over low heat. Add water and simmer for 2 hours. Season according to taste.

48. Clear Vegetable Broth

1 pt. hot vegetable stock
A little vegetable fat
Salt
Marmite or other yeast extract (opt.)
Chives or parsley

Pour hot vegetable stock over vegetable fat and herbs.

49. Tapioca Soup with Vegetables

1/2 oz. tapioca
1 pt. vegetable stock
1 tsp. vegetable fat
1 small carrot (opt.)
1 small piece of celeriac (opt.)
1/4 leek (opt.)
Salt

*Heat vegetable stock, and stir tapioca into it. Cut carrots and celeriac into small cubes and leek into small strips. Sauté vegetables in the fat, add to stock and cook for 15–20 minutes. If vegetables are omitted, add chives and vegetable fat before serving.

50. Clear Rice Soup

1/4 chopped onion
1 tbsp. finely chopped vegetables (carrots, celeriac and leeks)
1 tbsp. rice
1 pt. hot vegetable stock
Chives
1 tsp. vegetable fat

*Steam vegetables and rice in a little broth, add hot stock and cook for 15–20 minutes. Add chives and 1 tsp. vegetable fat before serving.

51. Thick Rice Soup

1 tsp. vegetable fat
1 piece celeriac
1 small, finely cut carrot
1/4 leek
1 level tbsp. rice
1 tsp. flour
1 pt. vegetable stock or water
Salt, chives

*Sauté vegetables and rice in fat, sprinkle with flour, add liquid and cook for 30 minutes. Add chives before serving.

52. Italian Rice Soup

1 tsp. vegetable fat
1 tbsp. finely diced vegetables (carrots, onions, and celery)
4 oz. spinach, finely cut
1 tbsp. rice
1 pt. water
Salt

*Sauté vegetables except spinach in fat until their color brightens. Add spinach, rice, water and salt and cook for 20 minutes. Add a little vegetable fat before serving.

53. Creamed Rice Soup

3 tbsp. rice flour
1 tsp. flour
1/4 cup milk
1 pt. vegetable stock
Salt
1 level tsp. vegetable fat
Chives to taste

Bring stock to a boil. Blend rice, flour and salt into a smooth cream. Add to the boiling stock. Cook for 1/2 hour. Put vegetable fat and chives into soup bowl and add soup.

54. Cream Soup

1 tsp. vegetable fat
2 level tbsp. whole-wheat flour
1 pt. vegetable stock
Salt, chives, nutmeg

Prepare as in recipe no. 53.

55. Herb Soup

Prepare Cream Soup, recipe no. 54, and add fresh or dried herbs such as lovage, basil, tarragon, etc. according to taste.

56. Soy Soup

1 tsp. vegetable fat
1/4 onion
1 tbsp. flour
1 tbsp. soy flour
1 tomato (peeled, diced)
1 pt. vegetable stock
Salt, nutmeg

*Blend flour and soy flour into a smooth paste and stir into the broth. Add tomato and salt and cook for 30 minutes. Put nutmeg into soup bowl and pour soup over it.

57. Cream of Rolled Oats Soup

1 tsp. vegetable fat
1 tsp. flour
2 tbsp. rolled oats
1 pt. vegetable stock
1 piece celeriac
Salt, chives if desired

Prepare as in recipe no. 53.

58. Rolled Oats Soup, plain

2 tbsp. rolled oats
1 pt. cold water
Salt if desired

Cook oats in water (possibly with a little salt) 30–40 minutes and pass through a strainer. Put 1 tsp. vegetable fat into the soup bowl and pour soup over it.

59. Oat Flour Soup

1 tsp. vegetable fat
2 tbsp. oat flour
1-1/2 cups vegetable stock
1/2 cup milk
Salt, chives

*Brown flour in fat, add stock, milk and salt and cook for 30 minutes. Put chives into soup bowl and add soup.

60. Oat Groats Soup

1 tsp. vegetable fat
2 tbsp. oat groats
1-1/2 cups water
1/2 cup milk
1 small piece celeriac
Salt
Marmite or other yeast extract

*Sauté groats lightly in fat, add water, milk, celery and salt and cook for 1 hour. Put yeast extract into the soup bowl and pour soup over it.

61. Spelt Soup

1/2 tsp. vegetable fat
1/4 leek, finely cut
1 piece cereriac, diced
1-1/2 tsp. spelt (whole or cracked)
1 pt. vegetable stock
Salt, lovage

*Soak spelt for 12 hours. Sauté leek and celery in fat. Add spelt and continue to sauté very lightly. Add vegetable stock, salt and lovage and cook for 1 to 1-1/2 hours. The soup may be passed through a sieve or run through the blender.

Note: Prepare spelt flour soup as in recipe no. 59.

62. Barley Soup

1 tsp. vegetable fat
1 tbsp. leek, carrots, and celery root (finely shredded)
1-1/2 tsp. barley
1-1/2 cups water
1/2 cup milk
Salt, nutmeg, chives

*Sauté vegetables lightly. Add barley, water, milk and salt and cook for 1 hour. Put nutmeg and chives into soup bowl before serving.

63. Barley Flour Soup

Prepare the same as recipe no. 59.

64. Farina Soup

1 tbsp. farina
1 pt. vegetable stock
Salt, nutmeg, chives

Add farina and salt to the boiling vegetable stock and cook for 1/2 hour. Put nutmeg and chives into soup bowl before serving.

65. Tomato Soup, I

(Without fat.)

4 ripe summer tomatoes
1 dash salt
1 dash sugar
1/4 cup hot vegetable stock

Dice tomatoes and bring to a quick boil, and strain. Add salt, sugar, vegetable stock, and serve.

66. Tomato Soup, II

1 tsp. vegetable fat
1 small carrot
1 small piece celeriac
1/4 leek
Some rosemary
2 tomatoes
1 tbsp. flour
1 pt. vegetable stock
Chives, salt

*Cut vegetables into small pieces and sauté well in fat. Sprinkle flour over the mixture. Slowly add vegetable stock, salt and cook for 10 minutes. Add chives and serve.

67. Carrot Soup

1 tsp. vegetable fat
2 sliced carrots
2 tbsp. flour

1-1/2 cups vegetable stock
1/2 cup milk
1/4 tsp. caraway seed
Celery leaves or lovage

*Sauté carrots in fat, sprinkle with flour and continue to sauté lightly. Add stock and milk and cook for 1/2 hour. Strain. Put caraway seeds, celery leaves or lovage into the soup bowl and add soup.

68. Spinach Soup

1 tsp. vegetable fat
2 tbsp. flour
1 small plateful chopped spinach
1-1/2 cups vegetable stock
1 plateful spinach
2 peppermint leaves
Nutmeg

*Sauté flour in fat. Add finely chopped spinach and sauté. Add vegetable stock and cook for 20 minutes. Run the remaining ingredients through blender, or chop finely (do not cook), and add to the ready soup. This soup can also be made with taro leaves.

69. Celeriac Soup

1 tsp. vegetable fat
1 small celery root, finely chopped
1 tbsp. flour
1 pt. vegetable stock
1 small piece bay leaf
Lovage, nutmeg

*Sauté celery root in fat, sprinkle with flour and continue to sauté. Add vegetable stock, salt, bay leaf and cook for 3/4 hour. Strain. Put lovage and nutmeg into the soup bowl and add soup.

70. Cauliflower Soup

1 tsp. vegetable fat
1 tbsp. flour
1/2 small cauliflower
1 pt. vegetable stock
Salt
1 small piece bay leaf
Pinch of basil
Some Marmite or other yeast extract

*Sauté flour in fat. Cook cauliflower florets separately. Cut uncooked stalks into small pieces and sauté with flour. Add vegetable stock, salt and bay leaf and cook for 3/4 hour. Strain. Put remaining ingredients with soup into the soup bowl.

71. Chervil Soup

1 diced potato
1 tsp. flour
1 pt. vegetable stock
1 scant tbsp. chopped chervil

*Sauté potato and flour in vegetable fat, add to stock and cook for 1/2 hour. Strain. Put chervil into the soup bowl and add soup.

72. Spring Soup

1 tbsp. flour
1-1/2 cups water or vegetable stock
Salt
1/4 onion
1 tender carrot
Small celery leaves
A few leaves of spinach
A few leaves of lovage, sorrel, nettle or dandelion
1/2 cup milk

*Blend flour into a smooth paste. Add to vegetable stock and cook for 1/2 hour. Add to soup, cover and let stand for a few minutes. Add milk and heat very briefly. Do not boil.

73. Potato Soup

1/2 leek
1 piece celeriac
1/2 carrot
1 large potato (diced)
1 level tbsp. flour
1 pt. water
A little vegetable stock
Salt, marjoram, chives

*Steam leek, celery, carrot and potato in vegetable stock. Sprinkle with flour. Add water and salt and cook for 1/2 hour. Strain. Put marjoram and chives into soup bowl, add soup.

74. Potato Soup with Leek

1/2 leek (cut into fine strips)
1 scant tbsp. flour
1 pt. vegetable stock
1 diced potato
Salt
Marmite or other yeast extract
Basil, marjoram, and other herbs

*Steam leek in a small amount of vegetable stock, sprinkle with flour. Add remaining stock, potato and salt and cook until tender. Put yeast extract and herbs into soup bowl and add soup.

75. Minestra

1/2 garlic clove
1 piece celery root
1/2 leek
2 celery leaves
1 small plateful of taro leaves
1 pt. water
Salt
1 tbsp. noodles or rice
1 pat of butter
Lovage or thyme

*Finely chop vegetables and garlic and steam in a little liquid. Add water, salt and cook for 1/2 hour. Add noodles or rice and cook for 15–20 minutes. Serve soup with butter, lovage or thyme.

Cooked Vegetables

Note for all recipes designated by an asterisk. For the liver patient's diet, we understand the term *steam* to mean the following: Turn vegetables in a small amount of non-fat vegetable stock. Use a tightly covered skillet. Add a little vegetable fat or oil to the ready dish before serving. Carefully avoid heating or browning of fats.

To preserve the nutritional value of cooked vegetables, the same basic rules apply for their preparation as were suggested for raw vegetables: cleanliness, freshness and careful preparation.

Almost all vegetables can be cooked in their own juice or in a little added vegetable stock. If vegetables have to be cooked in salted water, the water can be used later for sauces or soups. Only the water in which asparagus has been cooked is not wholesome and should be discarded.

If fresh vegetables are difficult to obtain, frozen ones may be used instead.

Cooking time, measures and weights for vegetables cannot always be given exactly since freshness and size often vary, as does the individual's appetite.

A few ingredients may be added or omitted, depending on taste.

It is very important to use very little salt. Salt can be replaced by the addition of subtly blended herbs. For sensitive patients, plainly cooked vegetables should be used, that is, cooked without any addition of fat.

The following vegetables are especially recommended for liver patients: Spinach, Romaine lettuce, endives, chicory, taro stalks, celery, fennel, carrots, peas, Chinese peas, celeriac, salsify, tomatoes, zucchini, pepper, cauliflower, kohlrabi, beets, artichokes, Jerusalem artichokes, eggplants.

These vegetables can all be prepared plainly in a little fat-free vegetable stock. Thereafter, they may be cut and served with herbs and possibly with onion juice.

76. Spinach, I

3/4 lb. spinach
A little vegetable stock
Salt, nutmeg, Marmite or other yeast extract

*Pick over spinach, remove thick stalks, wash and drain thoroughly. Steam whole leaves in covered pan with a very small amount of vegetable stock and salt over a low flame. Add nutmeg and Marmite or other yeast extract to taste.

Note: Overgrown winter spinach should be blanched briefly in salted water. Otherwise it may have a bitter taste.

77. Spinach, II

3/4 lb. spinach
1 tsp. pine kernels
1 tsp. raisins
A little water
Salt

*Prepare spinach as in recipe no. 76. Add raisins and salt and continue to steam briefly.

78. Spinach, III

3/4 lb. spinach
Salt
Peppermint leaves
Nutmeg
3/4 cup raw spinach

*Pick over spinach, and remove thick stalks. Wash thor-

oughly. Do not drain. Put spinach into pan, add salt and
steam covered over low flame until the water collects. Keep
water for later use. Mince or chop spinach. Season with
nutmeg and peppermint leaves. Chop raw spinach and add
to the cooked spinach.

79. Romaine Lettuce (steamed)

1 head Romaine lettuce
1 pt. salt water
1/4 cup vegetable stock

*Clean and halve lettuce, and cook in salt water until
nearly soft. Put into a colander to drain. Add vegetable
stock and simmer for about 20 minutes over low heat.

80. Steamed Endive

1 head endive
1 pt. salt water
1/4 cup vegetable stock

Prepare as in recipe no. 79.

81. Chicory

1/2 lb. chicory, prepared
2 tsp. milk
1/4 cup vegetable stock
Salt
Possibly a few drops of lemon juice

*Make crosswise incision in chicory stalks and put

chicory into saucepan in layers. Add milk, vegetable stock, and salt. Cover and steam over low flame for 1/4 hour. Add lemon juice if desired.

82. Taro Stalks

1/2 lb. taro stalks, prepared
Approximately 1/2 cup vegetable stock
Few drops of lemon juice
Salt

*Cut stalks into inch-long pieces and put into saucepan in layers. Add vegetable stock, lemon juice and salt. Cover and steam over a low flame for 1/2–3/4 hour until tender.

83. Celery

1/2 lb. celery
1/2 cup vegetable stock
A few drops lemon juice or 2 tbsp. milk
Salt

*Cut celery into 3-inch long pieces and put into skillet. Add vegetable stock, lemon juice or milk and salt. Cover and cook over low flame for 1/2–1 hour until tender.

84. Fennel

1 large or 2 small fennel
2 tbsp. milk
1/4 cup vegetable stock
Salt

*Cut fennel into halves, wash and cut out tough parts. Add milk, vegetable stock and salt. Cover and cook for 3/4 hour until tender.

85. Swiss Chard

1 small bunch of chard
1 pt. water
1/4 cup milk
Salt

Prepare chard and cut into finger-length pieces. Bring water, milk and salt to a boil. Add chard and cook for 1 hour or until tender.

86. Steamed Carrots

7 oz. carrots (3–4 carrots), cut into thin slices
1/2 cup vegetable stock
Salt, rosemary

*Steam carrots, vegetable stock and rosemary for 20–30 minutes.

87. Peas and Carrots

(Only sweet, young peas, if permitted and tolerated.)

4 oz. shelled peas
4 oz. carrots (prepared)
A little onion
1/2 cup vegetable stock (1/4 cup for each vegetable)
Pinch of sugar (for peas)

Prepare peas as in recipe no. 88. Cut carrots into small pieces and prepare according to recipe no. 86. Mix peas and carrots before serving, or arrange alternately on a serving dish.

88. Peas

(If permitted and tolerated.)

    1-1/2 cups very young, sweet peas (shelled)
    1/2 cup vegetable stock
    Salt, pinch of sugar

*Steam peas, vegetable stock, salt and sugar over a very low flame until peas are tender, depending on the quality of the peas, for 20–30 minutes.

89. Peas, French Style

(If permitted and tolerated.)

    1/4 head of Boston lettuce or Romaine (shredded into
        julienne strips)
    3/4 cup very young, sweet peas (shelled)
    1/4 cup vegetable stock
    Salt

*Steam lettuce briefly in its own juice. Add peas, vegetable stock and salt. Cook over very low flame until tender.

90. Chinese Peas

1 cup Chinese peas (prepared)
Salt, pinch of sugar
1/4 cup vegetable stock
Some parsley or lovage
1 scant tsp. cornstarch (opt.)

*Steam peas, salt and sugar in stock for 1/2–1 hour. Parsley or lovage may be cooked with the above or added as a garnish. Thicken juices with cornstarch, if desired.

91. Celeriac

8 oz. celery root (prepared)
A few drops lemon juice or 2 tbsp. milk
1/2 cup vegetable stock
Salt

*Cut celery root into small square slices. Add lemon juice or milk, vegetable stock and salt, cover and cook until tender for 1/2–3/4 hour.

92. Salsify

8 oz. salsify (prepared)
1/4 cup milk
1/2 cup vegetable stock
Salt

*Cut salsify into finger-length pieces. Add milk and vegetable stock, cover and cook over low flame for 3/4 hour.

93. Red Beets

6 oz. red beets
Salted water to cover
1 tsp. vegetable fat
1/4 cup vegetable stock
1 apple
A pinch of sugar
A few drops lemon juice
1 small bay leaf
A pinch of caraway seeds
Salt (if necessary)
Cornstarch (opt.)

*Cut the tips of roots and leaves to approximately 3/4 of an inch. Wash well without injuring the skin. Cook beets in salted water for 2–3 hours (or 25 minutes in a pressure cooker) until tender. Rinse them in cold water, peel and cut into fine slices. Bring to a boil equal parts of vegetable stock and the cooking water, adding caraway seeds, lemon juice, diced apple, cornstarch, sugar, bay leaf, salt, and the beets. Bring to a brief boil.

94. Jerusalem Artichokes

8 oz. Jerusalem artichokes
Salt
Water
A little vegetable stock
Basil

*Brush and wash Jerusalem artichokes. Use a trivet or wire basket to hold the vegetable just above the water in a saucepan. Add salt, cover and steam for 30–40 minutes.

Peel and slice Jerusalem artichokes and sauté them briefly in vegetable stock. Season with basil.

95. Steamed Tomatoes

6 oz. tomatoes
1/2 clove garlic
1 tsp. cornstarch (opt.)
Plenty of chopped parsley or other herbs

*Pour boiling water over the tomatoes and peel (very ripe tomatoes may be peeled without scalding). Put sliced tomatoes into a skillet, cover and steam gently in their own juice until they are somewhat reduced. Add garlic and cook until tender, possibly adding cornstarch for thickening. Sprinkle with parsley or other herbs.

96. Baked Tomatoes

6 oz. tomatoes
Salt
3/4 tbsp. vegetable fat

*Halve tomatoes and put in a greased baking dish. Sprinkle with salt. Put a dab of vegetable fat on each half and bake for about fifteen minutes in a moderate oven.

97. Filled Tomatoes

3 tomatoes
Salt
3 tsp. rice
1-1/2 tbsp. vegetable fat
Herbs (basil, thyme and rosemary)

Cut tops off tomatoes (save), and remove inside pulp. Chop pulp and mix with 1 tsp. uncooked rice per tomato. Add salt and herbs to taste. Fill tomatoes with mixture and put a dab of vegetable fat on each tomato. Cover with the tops, and put in a greased baking dish. Bake in a moderate oven for about 30 minutes.

98. Tomatoes à la Provencale

2 tomatoes
Salt
1 tbsp. parsley
Fine bread crumbs (1–2 tbsp.)

Halve tomatoes and sprinkle with salt. Put in a greased baking dish. Mix bread crumbs with chopped parsley and top tomatoes with mixture. Bake in a moderate oven.

99. Zucchini, I

8 oz. zucchini
Small pieces of vegetable fat
Salt
Rosemary, dill, parsley
Vegetable stock (opt.)

Select young, tender and small zucchini. Wash well. Cut off both ends. Cut in halves and put on a flat baking sheet. Cover with vegetable fat, salt, rosemary, dill and parsley and bake in a moderate oven. If necessary, add a little vegetable stock. Serve with Tomato Sauce, recipe no. 146.

100. Zucchini, II

8 oz. zucchini
Salt
Rosemary, dill, parsley
Vegetable stock (opt.)

*Dice zucchini (remove seeds of larger zucchini). Add salt, a little vegetable stock if needed, and steam covered until tender. Season with chopped herbs just before serving.

101. Zucchini, III

6 oz. zucchini
Fine breadcrumbs
Salt
Rosemary, dill, parsley
2–3 oz. tomatoes (approx.)

Halve zucchini and top with mixture of breadcrumbs, salt and herbs. Bake in moderate oven as in recipe no. 98. At the last, add peeled and diced tomatoes and steam briefly together with the zucchini. If excessive liquid forms, add cornstarch mixed with a little water, for thickening.

102. Peppers, Green or Yellow

(Peppers should be served as a side dish. Some liver patients do not tolerate them well.)

2 bell peppers
1/4 onion
Salt

*Cut peppers into strips and steam, covered, in a skillet with a small amount of vegetable stock for 20–30 minutes.

103. Mixed Vegetables

1 small zucchini
1/4 eggplant
1 tomato
Salt
1–2 small potatoes

*Halve zucchini, remove seeds of eggplant, and dice. Peel tomato and cut into large cubes. Season with salt. Dice potatoes and add to mixture. Steam, covered, for 1/2 hour. To reduce liquid, cook uncovered for a few minutes.

104. Eggplant

1 eggplant
Salt
Small amount vegetable stock

*Wash eggplant, peel and dice. Steam, covered, until tender. Garnish with Baked Tomatoes, recipe no. 96 or with Steamed Tomatoes, recipe no. 95.

105. Artichokes

1–2 artichokes
1 pt. water
Salt
1/2 tsp. lemon juice
Vinaigrette Sauce, no. 149

Cut off stems, remove hard lower leaves and cut off tips of other leaves. Halve artichokes and cut out choke. Wash under running water and sprinkle cut surfaces with lemon juice. Bring water and salt to a boil, add artichokes and cook until tender for about 3/4 hour. Drain, arrange on a hot dish covered with a napkin. Serve with Vinaigrette Sauce.

106. Steamed Artichoke Bottoms

  2–3 artichokes
  Salt
  A small amount of vegetable stock

*Cut out the soft artichoke bottoms, and rub them with lemon, sprinkle with salt and steam in vegetable stock until tender.

107. Corn on the Cob

(Chew very well, to facilitate digestion.)

  1–2 ears of corn
  1 pt. salted water
  Vegetable fat

Choose corn with tender, milky kernels. Shuck the ears and cook uncovered in salted water for 10 to 20 minutes. Serve on a hot plate covered with a napkin. Serve with vegetable fat or cottage cheese.

108. Cauliflower

(If permitted and tolerated.)

    1 small cauliflower
    1 pt. salted water

Cut off the stalks and leaves at the bottom and quarter the head. Peel stalks and keep tender leaves. Soak for one hour in cold salt water, rinse well. Cook cauliflower in salted water for 20–30 minutes. Serve on a hot, deep dish. Serve with a little softened (not heated) vegetable fat or some Tomato Sauce, recipe no. 147.

Cauliflower is the most easily digested of the cabbages and can therefore be eaten by patients suffering from gastric ailments.

109. Broccoli

(If permitted and tolerated.)

Prepare the same way as Cauliflower, recipe no. 108.

110. Kohlrabi

(If permitted and tolerated.)

    1–2 kohlrabi
    1/2–1 cup vegetable stock
    Salt
    Tender kohlrabi leaves, finely chopped

*Quarter kohlrabi, then slice finely. Add vegetable stock

and steam covered for 1/2 hour. Add salt and kohlrabi leaves just before serving.

Note: If tender kohlrabi leaves are not available, use chopped parsley. Very tender kohlrabi need only be quartered.

Cooked Vegetable Salads

Carrots, celeriac, beets, cauliflower, and Chinese artichokes are especially well suited for salads.

The vegetables are cooked in vegetable stock or salted water until tender. They can then be cut into small pieces (diced, sliced, etc.) and served with salad dressings. Use chopped herbs and onions for seasoning.

111. Mixed Vegetable Salad

Use 3–4 different varieties of cooked vegetables such as carrots, celeriac, cauliflower, Chinese artichokes, zucchini, beets and potatoes. Dice or slice vegetables and mix with salad dressings (recipes no. 7, 8).

112. Rice Salad

1 tbsp. rice
1-1/4 cups water
Salt
1 tbsp. oil
1 tsp. lemon juice
1 small tomato, finely chopped
1 small gherkin, finely chopped
A few capers
Chives, parsley, basil

Cook rice, strain and rinse through a sieve and let cool. Mix oil and lemon juice thoroughly and mix with rice. Mix all other ingredients with rice. Serve on lettuce leaves or in shells.

113. Vegetable Aspic

1 pt. vegetable stock (lukewarm)
1/4 tsp. Agar-Agar†
A few drops lemon juice
Marmite or other yeast extract
Salt
Tomato cubes
Gherkin
Cooked cauliflower
Cooked peas
Cooked green beans

Mix Agar-Agar in lukewarm vegetable stock and heat slowly until it is completely dissolved. Season with lemon juice, salt and yeast extract. Dice the vegetables.

Pour a little aspic into previously rinsed mold. Leave to set in a cool place. Garnish with vegetable cubes, pour in a little more aspic, and let set again. Repeat until the dish is filled. When aspic has set, turn over mold and garnish salad dishes with aspic.

Canapés and Sandwiches

Canapés or open-faced sandwiches are popular as hors d'oeuvres or an evening meal in the summertime, as well as for travel and hiking trips. Spreads can be varied and com-

---

† Agar-Agar is a vegetable gelatine made from seaweed. Available as a powder in health food stores, it can be used instead of gelatine for vegetables, fruits, sauces and puddings.

bined in many ways. The fresher and more colorful the slices look, the more appetizing they will be. Use whole-grain rye bread and pumpernickel. Whole-wheat bread should be at least one day old so that it can be cut into thin slices.

114. Basic Spreads

Cottage cheese or vegetable fat
Salt, yeast extract, chives, herbs, caraway seeds, or
    tomato purée

Mix all ingredients into the cottage cheese or the vegetable fat. Garnish with raw grated carrots or celery, tomatoes, radishes, cress, gherkins, capers, olives, etc.

Potato Dishes

115. Potatoes in Their Skins

(Yellow and red potatoes are especially well suited.)

8 oz. potatoes
Salt
Water

Brush potatoes and wash. Steam in a special steamer or in a wire basket fitted into a saucepan. Fill with salted water up to the basket, cover and steam for 30–40 minutes. Follow the directions of the pressure cooker when using one.

116. Baked Potatoes

8 oz. potatoes (medium-sized)
Salt
1–1-1/2 tsp. oil

Brush potatoes. Wash well. Score skin on upper part 3–4 times. Brush with oil and salt. Bake on a greased baking sheet for 30–40 minutes in medium heat. Put a dab of vegetable fat on each potato before serving (if permitted).

117. Potatoes with Cottage Cheese

8 oz. potatoes
Salt
1–1-1/2 tsp. oil

FILLING:

1/4 cup cottage cheese (low-fat or regular)
1 tbsp. milk
1 dash of salt
Chives, caraway seeds or marjoram

Brush potatoes and wash well. Score once across upper part of potato. Brush with oil, add salt and bake for 30–40 minutes in moderate oven. Whip cottage cheese with milk, mix in other ingredients. Put into a pastry bag and pipe over the slit of the baked potatoes.

118. Caraway Potatoes

2–3 medium potatoes
A few caraway seeds
Salt, oil

Brush potatoes and wash well. Halve potatoes crosswise. Mix caraway seeds and salt and dip the cut side of the potatoes into the mixture. Place on a slightly greased baking sheet, cut surfaces down. Bake for 45 minutes in moderate oven.

119. Bouillon Potatoes

8 oz. potatoes
1-1-1/4 cups slightly salted vegetable stock

Wash and peel potatoes, halve or slice them and cook in vegetable stock until tender. Melt a small amount of vegetable fat over potatoes before serving (if permitted).

120. Parsley Potatoes

8 oz. potatoes (peeled)
Salt
A small amount of water
1 tsp. parsley (chopped)

Cut potatoes lengthwise into four pieces. Sprinkle with salt. Steam potatoes in a wire basket over boiling water. Melt vegetable fat (if permitted), mix with parsley and potatoes and serve.

121. Cream Potatoes

6–7 oz potatoes (peeled)
1 cup vegetable stock
Salt
1/4 cup buttermilk or low-fat milk
Parsley

Cut potatoes into slices. Steam briefly and cook until tender in vegetable stock and milk. Before serving sprinkle with parsley.

122. Potatoes with Tomatoes

6–7 oz. potatoes
3/4 cup vegetable stock
Salt
3–4 oz. tomatoes

Peel potatoes, cut into slices and cook gently in stock. Peel tomatoes, dice and add to potatoes just before they are done.

123. Potato Snow

8 oz. potatoes
Salt, water

Peel potatoes, slice and steam in a little water until tender. Force hot, cooked potatoes through a sieve directly onto a warm dish. Add a few dabs of vegetable fat (if permitted).

124. Mashed Potatoes

8 oz. potatoes
A little water
Salt
1 tbsp. vegetable fat
1/2–3/4 cup milk or buttermilk or low-fat milk
Nutmeg

Peel potatoes, slice and steam in a little water until tender. Force potatoes through a sieve. Warm vegetable fat and milk, add potatoes and mash thoroughly. Season with nutmeg. Serve on a hot dish. Use a hot knife to make attractive patterns.

Grain Dishes

Note for all recipes designated by an asterisk: Turn vegetables briefly in a little nonfat vegetable stock. Pour a little vegetable fat on the prepared vegetables. Carefully avoid all heating and browning of fat. For liver patients do not sauté in oil any of the rice dishes. Instead add rice directly to the boiling vegetable stock. Brown rice should be cooked, covered, for 40 minutes without stirring, white rice for 12–15 minutes (less in a pressure cooker). Brown rice is used for all rice dishes except desserts.

125. Japanese Rice

1/4–1/2 cup brown rice
3/4–1 cup water
Salt
3/4 tbsp. vegetable fat

*Put rice into boiling water or vegetable stock and cook for 40 minutes. Rice should be grainy. Permit to cool. Warm rice on a baking sheet in an oven and put dabs of vegetable fat on it before serving (if permitted).

126. Rice Creole

1/4–1/2 cup brown rice
3/4–1 cup water or vegetable stock
Salt

*Put rice into boiling water or vegetable stock and cook for 40 minutes or until liquid is absorbed.

127. Rice Creole with Vegetables

1/2 cup finely chopped celeriac and carrots
1/4–1/2 cup brown rice
3/4–1 cup vegetable stock
Salt

*Put rice and vegetables into boiling vegetable stock and cook until liquid is absorbed.

128. Rice with Tomatoes

1/4–1/2 cup brown rice
2 small tomatoes
Salt
3/4–1 cup vegetable stock

*Peel tomatoes, dice and add with salt to the rice. Add vegetable stock and cook until liquid is absorbed.

129. Rice with Zucchini

3 oz. young zucchini
Oil
1/4 cup vegetable stock or water
1/4–1/2 cup brown rice

*Dice zucchini and sauté briefly in oil. Slowly add vegetable stock or water and rice and cook until a risotto is formed.

130. Rice with Peas

1/2–3/4 cup shelled peas
Oil
1/2 cup vegetable stock
1/4–1/2 cup brown rice
1 cup water
Salt

Briefly sauté peas in oil. Thereafter, cook until tender in vegetable stock. Prepare Rice Creole or Japanese Rice (recipes no. 126, 125). Add cooked peas to the prepared rice.

131. Rice with Spinach

1/4 cup coarsely chopped spinach
1/4–1/2 cup brown rice
Oil
1 cup hot water or vegetable stock

*Sauté spinach and rice. Add water or vegetable stock and cook until liquid is absorbed.

132. Rice Ring or Pudding

Put Japanese Rice or Rice Creole into a ring mold or cups rinsed in cold water. Turn out onto a dish.

Rice Ring: Fill center with steamed tomatoes or steamed peas and carrots.

Rice Pudding: Garnish with sautéed tomato slices.

Small Rice Pudding: Garnish with baked tomato halves.

133. Farina Pudding

1-1/2 oz. farina
1 cup milk (whole or low-fat)
1/4 cup water
Salt

Bring milk, water and salt to a boil. Add farina, stirring all the time. Cook for 15–20 minutes.

134. Farina Balls

2 oz. farina
1 cup milk (whole or low-fat)
1/4 cup water
Salt

Bring milk, water and salt to a boil. Add farina, stirring all the time. Dip a small ladle into the boiling water and scoop out small balls of farina.

135. Corn Mash

2 oz. yellow cornmeal
1 tbsp. farina
3/4 cup milk (whole or low-fat)
1-1/4 cups water
Salt
A little vegetable fat

Stir cornmeal, farina and salt into the boiling liquid. Cook for 5 minutes over medium-high heat while continuously stirring. Then cook on low heat for another hour, stirring occasionally. Add dabs of vegetable fat to the finished dish (if permitted).

136. Polenta

1 tsp. oil
1-1/4–2 oz. yellow cornmeal
1-3/4 cups water
Salt
Nutmeg

Coat saucepan with oil, add water and bring to a boil. Stir in cornmeal, salt and nutmeg and cook for 5 minutes over high heat, stirring continuously. Then cook slowly for another hour.

137. Millotto

2 oz. millet
5–6 oz. hot vegetable stock
Salt

*Bring vegetable stock and salt to a boil. Pour over millet and continue to cook for 20 minutes.

138. Millotto with Vegetables

1/2 cup diced vegetables (celeriac, carrots or carrots
   and peas)
1-1/4 oz. millet
Rosemary
5–6 oz. vegetable stock
Salt
3/4 tbsp. vegetable fat

*Cook diced vegetables, millet and rosemary in vegetable stock for 20 minutes. Add dabs of vegetable fat over finished dish.

139. Buckwheat

1/2 cup buckwheat (Ala)
1 cup water
Salt
3/4 tbsp. vegetable fat

Soak buckwheat for 24 hours. Steam in tightly covered pan for 1 hour. Serve with cold milk, yogurt or buttermilk. Add a little honey or vegetable fat (if permitted).

140. Whole-Wheat Porridge

1–1-1/2 oz. whole-wheat grains
1 tsp. ground millet (for thickening)

1-1/2 cups vegetable stock or half milk and half water
Salt
Fresh vegetable fat

Wash and dry wheat. Grind coarsely in coffee grinder or blender. Bring liquid to a boil. Stir in cereals and continue to cook for 30–40 minutes. Add dabs of vegetable fat to finished dish (if permitted).

141. Groat Porridge

4 tsp. crushed grains
6 tsp. water
Salt

Soak crushed grains in 1 tsp. water for 24 hours. Add 5 tsp. water and salt to the soaked cereal and cook for 10 minutes in a saucepan or for 1/2 hour in a double boiler.

142. Sweet Whole-Wheat Porridge

1–1-1/2 oz. whole-wheat grains
1 tbsp. farina or ground millet
1–1-1/4 cups milk (whole or low-fat)
Salt
1 tsp. honey
1 tsp. raisins (opt.)

Prepare the same as in recipe no. 140. Bring milk to a boil. Stir in cereals and cook until soft for 30–40 minutes. Serve with raisins and honey.

143. Spaghetti, Macaroni, Noodles

(Use dough prepared without eggs.)

2–3 oz. spaghetti, macaroni or noodles
1 pt. water (boiling)
Salt
Tomato Sauce no. 146

Cook macaroni, spaghetti or noodles in salt water for 15–20 minutes. Drain through a sieve. Rinse in cold water. Add Tomato Sauce before serving.

144. Noodles with Sage

2–3 oz. noodles
1 pt. water
Salt
1 fresh sage leaf
Basil, garlic
3/4 tbsp. vegetable fat

Cook noodles in salt water. Chop sage leaf, basil, and garlic, warm in melted vegetable fat and mix with noodles.

145. Soy Spaetzli

2 oz. whole-wheat flour
2 oz. soy flour
1/2–1 cup water
Salt
3/4 tbsp. vegetable fat

Mix whole-wheat flour, soy flour, a little water and salt. Beat and knead the dough well until bubbles form. Put aside for at least 1 hour. Bring salted water to a boil. Force batter, a small portion at a time, through a colander or grater with large perforations into the boiling water. Simmer until Spaetzli rise to surface. Take out with a perforated ladle and arrange on a hot dish. Add dabs of vegetable fat (if permitted). Instead of a sieve, one can use a wet wooden board on which the dough can be cut into fine strips, and dropped into the boiling water. The Spaetzli can also be cooked in vegetable stock and served immediately on a hot plate. This method assures more easily digestible Spaetzli.

Sauces

146. Tomato Sauce, I

A little garlic
2–3 peeled tomatoes
Salt
Basil, rosemary or thyme

*Dice tomatoes and sauté together with the other ingredients, in oil if permitted, or in their own juice.

147. Tomato Sauce, II

2–3 tomatoes
Salt
Rosemary, basil or thyme
1 tbsp. milk

*Slice tomatoes. Sauté gently (in oil if permitted) until tender and pass through a sieve. Add milk.

148. Carrot Sauce

1 medium carrot
1/2 cup vegetable stock
1 tsp. cream (if permitted)
1 dash salt
Possibly a little onion and rosemary

Mix all ingredients in a blender.

149. Vinaigrette

1 tbsp. olive oil
1 tsp. lemon juice
1 tsp. water or vegetable stock
1 tsp. chopped onions
1–2 minced gherkins
Parsley or chives
1 tsp. diced tomatoes
Salt

Whisk all ingredients together.

Desserts

150. Fruit in Syrup

Light corn syrup, honey or pure fruit syrup
1/2 cup water, *or*
1/4 cup water and 1/4 cup grape juice
7 oz. fresh, ripe apricots or peaches or plums

Dissolve syrup or honey in water and grape juice and bring to a boil. Halve fruit and remove stones. Cook briefly in the syrup. Cool. Serve on an attractive dish.

Note: When using strawberries, raspberries, blueberries or currants (black 1/3, red 2/3), pour boiling syrup over fruit.

151. Strawberries with Lemon Juice

7 oz. hulled strawberries
1/2 lemon
1 tbsp. sugar (fruit sugar if available)

Halve large strawberries. Add sugar and lemon juice.

152. Fruit Salad

A little honey
1/4 cup water
1/4–1/2 cup grape juice or apple cider
1 tsp. lemon juice
7 oz. mixed, ripe fruit (apricots or peaches, melons, apples, soft pears, red pitted cherries, any kind of berries)

Bring honey, water and juice or cider to a boil. Let it cool. Add lemon juice. Prepare a selection of fruits in season. Cut fruits into small slices and add to the cooled syrup.

153. Stuffed Melon

1 small melon
Fruit Salad no. 152

Halve melon and remove seeds. Fill with Fruit Salad.

154. Fruit Jello

1/2 cup water or grape juice
A little honey
1/4 tsp. Agar-Agar†
3/4 cup fruit juice (orange, berries)

Heat water or grape juice over low flame, adding Agar-Agar and sugar. Stir continuously until Agar-Agar is completely dissolved. Mix in fruit juice, cool and pour immediately into glasses or small dishes.

155. Apple Sauce

7 oz. apples
1/4 cup water or apple juice
A little lemon peel (opt.)
A little honey
Cinnamon

Remove cores, peel and cut apples into slices. Cook until tender. Put through a sieve. Add honey and cinnamon.

† See page 98.

156. Stewed Apples

7 oz. apples
1/2–3/4 cup water or apple juice
A little honey
lemon peel (grated) or a little cinnamon

Peel apples, remove cores and slice apples. Bring liquid to a boil. Add honey and cook apples until tender.

157. Apple Halves

2 apples
1/2–3/4 cup water or apple juice
A little honey
1 stick cinnamon
Quince, raspberry or currant jelly

Peel apples, halve and remove cores. Bring juice to a boil. Add apples and cook slowly until tender. Remove with perforated ladle and put on a dish, cut surfaces up. Fill apples with jelly.

158. Blueberry Sweet

8 oz. blueberries
1–2 oz. honey
1/4 cup water
1 level tsp. flour
1 tbsp. water

Wash blueberries and remove spoiled ones. Cook in honey and water for 5–10 minutes. Blend flour with water. Add to blueberries and bring to a boil. Serve.

159. Stewed Rhubarb

8 oz. rhubarb
1-1/2–2 oz. honey
1/4 cup water
Cornstarch for thickening

Wash rhubarb and cut into small pieces. Cook in honey and water until tender. Remove rhubarb with perforated ladle. Boil down juice to thicken, or add cornstarch, and pour over rhubarb. Some liver patients do not tolerate rhubarb.

160. Stuffed Apples

2 medium apples
2 tsp. ground almonds
1 tsp. currants
1 tbsp. sweetened condensed milk
1–2 tsp. honey
A little lemon peel (grated)
1 dab butter
1 tsp. sugar
1/4 cup apple juice

Remove apple cores and make an incision into the skin. Mix nuts, currants, milk, honey, lemon peel and fill center of apples with mixture. Put apples into a baking dish. Put a small dab of butter and 1/2 tsp. sugar over each apple and fill dish with apple juice to about 1/2 inch. Bake in oven for 20–30 minutes.

Use recipe only if almonds are tolerated.

161. Lemon Whip

1 cup water
1/2 lemon
1 tsp. cornstarch
1 tbsp. milk
1–2 tbsp. honey

Peel lemon very thinly and bring peel to a boil in the water. Mix cornstarch with cold milk, add fruit sugar and add to the boiling water. Bring again to a boil. Cool, then strain. Add a little lemon juice.

162. Orange Molds

3/4 cup orange juice
1/8 tsp. Agar-Agar†
1 tsp. sugar or honey

Whisk Agar-Agar and honey or sugar into 1/2 cup orange juice over low flame. Do not bring to a boil. Continue until Agar-Agar is completely dissolved. Add remainder of orange juice and pour into previously rinsed, cold molds. Refrigerate.

163. Almond Milk Sauce

1/2 cup milk
1/2 oz. almonds (peeled and grated), *or* almond purée
1/2 oz. honey or sugar
1 tsp. cornstarch
1 tbsp. water

† See page 98.

Bring milk, almonds or almond purée and sugar to a boil. Mix cornstarch with water and add to the boiling milk. Put into blender or strain through a sieve.

164. Rose Hip Sauce

3/4 oz. rose hip purée
1/4 cup water or grape juice
A little honey
A few drops lemon juice (opt.)

Bring rose hip purée, water, juice and honey to a boil. Add lemon juice.

164a. Rose Hip Purée

2 oz. dried rose hips
3/4–1 cup boiling water
1 oz. sugar or honey

Bring rose hips and water to a boil and simmer for 15 minutes. Boil sugar or honey in 1–2 tbsp. water until it becomes syrupy. Mix with mashed hips and boil for 10 minutes.

165. Red Wine Sauce

1/4 cup water
Lemon or orange peel
1/4 stick cinnamon
1 clove
A little honey or sugar
1/4 cup grape juice
1 tsp. almonds

Bring water, lemon or orange peel, cinnamon, clove and honey to a boil. Cook for a few minutes. Strain and add grape juice. Heat again, but do not boil. Peel almonds, cut into slivers and add to sauce.

166. Punch (Nonalcoholic)

1/2 cup water
1/2 cup apple cider
1/2 cup grape juice
1 slice of lemon
1 small piece cinnamon
1 clove
1 tbsp. honey
1 tsp. lemon juice
1 tbsp. fruit syrup

Boil water, lemon and spices for 5 minutes. Strain and add cider and grape juice. Heat again and add lemon juice, honey and syrup. Serve hot.

167. Farina Pudding

1-1/2 oz. farina
1-1/2–2 cups whole milk, water or low-fat milk
1 dash salt
1–2 tsp. sugar or honey
1 small piece of lemon peel (grated)
2 tsp. peeled and grated almonds
1/2 oz. raisins
Raspberry syrup

Boil liquid and add farina, stirring all the time. Add salt and lemon peel and cook for 15–20 minutes. Add sugar. Mix almonds and raisins with cooked farina. Pour into a previously rinsed mold. Serve with raspberry syrup or with sweetened, fresh berry juice thickened with cornstarch.

168. Rice Pudding with Steamed Fruit

2-1/2–3 oz. white rice
3/4 cup water
1 small piece of lemon peel (grated)
1 dash salt
1/2–3/4 cup hot milk (whole or low-fat)
1 tbsp. honey
1 tsp. vegetable fat

Bring water to a boil and add rice, lemon peel and salt. Cook for 15 minutes. Add honey and milk and continue to cook until rice is tender. Add fat and fill pudding into a rinsed mold. Turn out when cooled and garnish with steamed fruit.

Herb Teas

Herb teas are particularly recommended for liver patients.

169. Bitter Tea

Wormwood, Centaury and Blessed Thistle (in equal parts)

Pour boiling water over herbs and allow to steep for 5 minutes. To stimulate appetite, sip 2–3 tbsp., 1/2 hour before meals (mild cholagogue, i.e., increases flow of bile). For sensitive individuals: only Centaury.

170. Linseed Tea

1 tbsp. linseed
1 pt. water

Boil for 7–10 minutes and allow to steep a little. Mucolytic, mildly purgative.

171. Rose Hip Tea

2–3 tbsp. dried rose hips
1-1/2 qt. water

Soak rose hips for 12 hours. Simmer for 1/2–3/4 hour. Strain. Mildly cholagogue and diuretic.

172. Peppermint Tea

Pour boiling water over dried peppermint leaves. Allow to steep for a short time. Drink 2–3 cups per day. Cholagogue and sedative.

173. Wormwood Tea

Pour boiling water over wormwood and steep for 5 minutes. Strong Bitter tea, strongly stimulates the flow of bile and gastric juices. To be taken during the day in sips.

174. Seed Tea

Caraway, fennel and anise (in equal parts)

Pour boiling water over seeds and allow to steep for 20 minutes. Drink 1 cup after meals in case of flatulence.

Other Drinks. Mineral waters (consult physician); buttermilk (between meals); fresh fruit and vegetable juices.

Modern Kitchen Management

It is of great importance to preserve the full nutritional value of foods when preparing a patient's diet. Thoughtful selection and proper, careful preparation are mandatory. This will assure that the patient receives sufficient nutritive value as well as adequate amounts of vitamins, mineral substances, trace elements, enzymes and growth substances (auxins).

Below are given a few hints from our health-food kitchen. Particular attention should be paid to the quality of foods when shopping. Fruits, vegetables and potatoes should be organically grown to avoid loss in nutritional value due to the one-sided usage of artificial fertilizers and poisonous insecticides.

For the selection and treatment of vegetables and salads, based on our experience at the Bircher-Benner clinic, see pages 54-57 of this booklet.

To preserve valuable proteins and mineral salts, which are concentrated just below the skin, potatoes should be steamed in their skin and then peeled very thinly. Organically grown potatoes may also be eaten with the skin.

The practice of boiling vegetables and pouring out the cooking water is no longer advised. Vegetables, if not eaten raw or in salads, should be steamed or stewed in order to preserve the water-soluble mineral salts.

To steam a vegetable is to cook it in its own juice on low heat. This should be done in a steamer or in a skillet with a tight-fitting lid. An asbestos mat should be placed under the pan. Vegetables without much juice of their own need a little additional water after the initial steaming. This method insures abundant aroma and flavor and contributes to tastier dishes. The need for seasoning is kept to a minimum. In addition to vegetables, potato and rice dishes can also be steamed.

Steaming with additional water is necessary primarily in the preparation of potatoes. A small steaming device or a wire basket is inserted into a deep pot without touching the boiling water underneath.

A double boiler, or a tiered steaming pan,† circulates steam evenly around the food without dissolving valuable substances in the water. The vegetables are gently cooked in their own juices and retain their fresh color, aroma and nutritive value.

If possible, foods should not be kept warm for prolonged periods or reheated because of the loss in nutritive value. According to the latest findings, reheating food once is less damaging than keeping it warm.

In addition to steamers and steaming inserts, the following items should be on hand: A glass or chrome-plated two-way grater for fine and coarse grating of fruits and vegetables. A nut mill for the often used nuts and almonds. A hand mill for coarse grinding of grains. An electric blender to chop, grind, grate and blend raw foods. A juice extractor for the preparation of vegetable and fruit juices. For very large quantities, a hydraulic juice extractor may be helpful.

Seasoning enlivens a dish and makes it interesting, palatable and appetizing. Correct seasoning is an art which requires experience.

---

† The steamers, available at Chinese markets in this country, allow steaming of several dishes at once.—ED.

One should be very careful with the use of salt and strong, tropical spices particularly when preparing a patient's diet. Since steaming and sautéing preserve the original taste of the food, very little seasoning is required. Many nuances of taste are offered by the great variety of local herbs available throughout the year. These are generally added just before serving a dish.

Also recommended for seasoning are yeast extracts, and sea salt instead of regular cooking salt.

In conclusion, the importance of good, slow chewing should be pointed out.